Markets and Health Care: A Comparative Analysis

Edited by Wendy Ranade

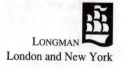

LONGMAN
London and New York

Addison Wesley Longman Limited
Edinburgh Gate
Harlow
Essex CM20 2JE
United Kingdom
and Associated Companies throughout the world

Published in the United States of America by Addison Wesley Longman, New York

First published 1998

ISBN 0 582 28985 8

British Library Cataloguing-in-Publication Data

A catalogue record for this book is available from the British Library

Library of Congress Cataloging-in-Publication Data

Markets and health care: a comparative analysis / edited by Wendy Ranade.
p. cm.
Includes bibliographical references and index.
ISBN 0-582-28985-8 (pbk.: alk. paper)
1. Medical care—Finance. 2. Competition. 3. Health care reform—Case studies. I.
Ranade, Wendy, 1940–.
RA411.M36 1998
338.4'33621—dc21

97-37202
CIP

Set by 7 in 10/11pt Times
Produced through Longman Malaysia, PA

CONTENTS

THE CONTRIBUTORS

John Appleby is Senior Lecturer in Health Economics at the University of East Anglia. He worked in the National Health Service for seven years, helping to set up an information department in South Birmingham Health Authority and later becoming manager of the National Association of Health Authorities Central Policy Unit. John has published widely on a range of health care finance and economic issues and his current research interests include the opportunity cost of inappropriate health care, the use of economic evaluation and advice to health authorities, the measurement of competition and the macroeconomic issues of health service funding.

Pat Baranek is currently a PhD candidate in the Department of Health Administration at the University of Toronto. She has worked as a Manager of Policy in the Ontario provincial government in the areas of health, intergovernmental affairs, and citizenship. Pat's interests lie in the public/private mix in the financing of health care and policy issues involved in long-term care. She has also conducted and published research on the criminal justice system in Canada.

Jacqueline Cumming is a Research Fellow at the Victoria University of Wellington. She has worked for seven years as a policy analyst and economist in the health sector where she has concentrated on issues such as healthy communities, smokefree environment legislation and strategic health policy. Jacqueline has a wide knowledge of health economics and health policy and is experienced in the application of economic ideas and techniques to the development of health sector policies and strategies. She is currently researching the development of explicit packages of health care services and identifying public policy issues that arise in defining an explicit core of health services.

Raisa Deber is Professor in the Department of Health Administration at the University of Toronto. She is President of the Canadian Health Economics Research Association and is involved with the Society for the Medical Decision Making. Raisa teaches, researches and acts as a consultant on Canadian health policy.

Richard Freeman is Lecturer in European Policy and Politics at the

University of Edinburgh. His research interests lie in health policy and politics in Europe and in comparative social policy. He has written on the politics of prevention in health policy and on HIV and AIDS, and is currently completing a book on health politics in Europe. He is co-convenor of the ESRC research seminar on Welfare and Culture in Europe.

Professor Theodore Marmor is Professor of Public Policy and Political Science at the Yale School of Management, Yale University. He has played a leading part in debates on health care reform both nationally and internationally, and has acted as an advisor to a number of administrations in the U.S., including the Clinton administration. Professor Marmor has written extensively on health care policy and management as well as the politics and economics of the modern welfare state. His latest book is *Understanding Health Care Reform* published in 1994.

Michael Moran is Professor of Government at the University of Manchester. He has written books on British politics, the regulation of financial markets and the regulation of the medical profession. His chapter in this volume is part of a continuing project on governing the health care state.

Wendy Ranade retired as Reader in Government and Politics at the University of Northumbria at Newcastle in June 1997, and is now an Honorary Research Fellow as well as Chair of the Royal Victoria Infirmary and Associated Hospitals NHS Trust. She was a member and then Vice-Chair of Newcastle Health Authority from 1985–1992. Her main research interests are health policy and management and she has taught, researched and written widely in these fields. Her most recent book is the second edition of *A Future of the NHS?*, published by Addison Wesley Longman in 1997.

Ray Robinson is Professor of Health Policy and Director of the Institute for Health Policy Studies at the University of Southampton. He has worked as an economist in Her Majesty's Treasury, been Deputy Director of the King's Fund Institute and has acted as a consultant to health authorities, government departments and international organisations. He was also vice-chairman of East Sussex Health Authority. Ray's research interests include various aspects of health finance, economics and management and he has published widely in this field.

George Salmond is a University of Otago medical graduate and has trained as a physician, researcher and public health specialist. He directed the health services and research and planning units at the Department of Health in Wellington. In 1986 he was appointed Director-General of Health. He resigned in 1991 and then worked in

New Zealand and internationally as a public health consultant. In 1993 Professor Salmond became head of a Health Research Council of New Zealand funded Health Research Centre. His areas of interest and expertise are health sector management, health services research and development, public health practice and community health development.

Richard B. Saltman is Professor of Health Policy and Management at the Emory University School of Public Health in Atlanta, Georgia. He is also Visiting Professor in the Braun School of Public Health of Hadassah Medical School at Hebrew University in Jerusalem. He was co-project leader for the World Health Organisation/European Regional Office's 1995–96 study of health care reforms and has also been a consultant to health systems reform projects for the Organisation for Economic Cooperation and Development and the World Bank. His research focuses on the behaviour of European health care systems, particularly in the Nordic Region.

CHAPTER 1

Introduction

WENDY RANADE

This book starts with a paradox. Put crudely, in the study of health policy the United States has always been seen as a failure. While other Western democracies managed to combine a reasonably accessible and equitable system of health care for all their populations at an affordable cost to the nation, the United States – which alone of all the democracies still had a system based largely on private markets – combined the most expensive system in the world with millions of citizens uninsured or inadequately insured. As Moran puts it in Chapter 2, learning health policy lessons from the United States is rather like taking lessons in seamanship from the crew of the *Titanic*. Economic theory and practical experience seemed to combine to tell a forceful lesson: keep markets out of health care. Yet in the flurry of health care reform and restructuring that has characterised the 1990s the USA has gone from policy laggard to policy leader, the source of many of the ideas which underpin reforms elsewhere and in particular the introduction or strengthening of market principles in health care. The central point of our enquiry in this book is to try to answer the questions: why did this happen, and with what results?

A subtheme of the enquiry is the way in which policy learning and 'lesson drawing' between states takes place in an increasingly interdependent, information-rich world. Marmor (1995) observes that most policy debates in most countries are parochial affairs, rooted in national experience and developments, reflecting national political struggles and conflicting visions of the future. If (rarely) policy makers seriously look to foreign experience for solutions to problems it is used mainly as a tool of policy warfare in internal struggles, not policy understanding and careful lesson drawing. The international spread of promarket, procompetitive ideas in health care reform has involved more than its fair share of myth-making, distortion and the selective use of evidence from other countries.

The book brings together an international group of health policy analysts with different disciplinary backgrounds: political science, health economics, public health and public management. Though each chapter reflects the disciplinary perspective of its author(s), the group benefited from a three-day colloquium held at the Longhirst campus of the University of Northumbria in Newcastle in July 1996 which enabled early drafts to be thoroughly debated and exposed to different disciplinary foci. Michael Hill, Professor of Social Policy at the University of

Newcastle upon Tyne, attended the colloquium throughout the three days, and I would like gratefully to acknowledge his generosity in doing so, his contributions to the debate and his helpful comments on individual chapters. This sharing of ideas and perspectives enabled a richer analysis of complex and multifaceted phenomena to take place. The introductory chapter discusses some of the manifestations of the rise of the market in health care, clarifies some of the concepts and terms used throughout the book, briefly discusses some of the pitfalls of comparative analysis, sets out the contents and scope, and the rationale for the selection of countries examined.

The rise of the market in health care

What a market means in economic theory is discussed at length in Chapter 3, but all markets are also social constructions governed by formal and informal sets of rules and patterns of normative relationships. The core elements of any market are a structure of buyers and sellers, trading goods or services for money. Markets may be more or less competitive, more or less 'free' or subject to regulation by the state or other bodies (e.g. professional or industry associations).

Real health systems are more complex than the crude stereotypes used to describe them (as employed in the opening paragraph), and cannot be adequately described by a state–market or public–private dichotomy. For example, although the British look to the USA as the example par excellence of the market system, over 40 per cent of health spending there passes through government hands, either federal or state (mainly for the financing and administration of Medicare for the elderly, and Medicaid for the indigent) (Newhouse, 1996). Conversely, the American public regard the British National Health Service (NHS) as a prime example of 'socialised medicine' almost akin to the centralised systems of the former Soviet Union, yet at least 52 per cent of health spending by the NHS takes place in the private sector (Salter, 1995). All health systems are a mixture of public and private elements: the rise of the market in health care involves an incremental shift and the selected application of various market 'tools' or instruments to different parts of the health system, rather than a wholesale move from one kind of system to another.

For example, most countries use a combination of different methods to finance health care, but three main methods predominate:

- public finance through general taxation (the 'Beveridge model') used by the UK, New Zealand, the Nordic countries, Canada, Italy and Spain;
- public finance through compulsory social insurance (the 'Bismarck model') used in Germany, the Netherlands, France and Belgium;

- private finance based on voluntary insurance or direct payments, largely used in the USA.

The extent to which the first two methods are supplemented by direct charges or private payments differs considerably from one country to another, but one sign of the rise of the market is the increasing use of co-payments or charges levied on patients. This may be coupled with tighter definitions of what will be provided by the public system, and what will be excluded. In the supposedly 'free' health systems of Europe about 80 million people have supplementary health insurance to cover them for services not provided by the public scheme or to pay for these out-of-pocket expenses (Moran, 1994).

Once the funds for health care are raised, they are reallocated to providers, again by a variety of methods. Given the uncertainty and risks associated with health care – people cannot predict when they will need services and the costs may be very high – the industry is a prime candidate for some form of insurance. The use of intermediaries to bear the financial risks involved, and act as third party payers to providers on behalf of their insured population, is therefore widespread (this is discussed in greater detail in Chapter 3). Who undertakes this role, and the 'risk pools' covered varies considerably: it may be national or regional governments, government appointed bodies, voluntary or charitable organisations or private insurance companies. A useful way to categorise the variety of payment methods in the OECD countries is the classification provided by Hurst (1992), and is shown in a simplified diagrammatic form in Figure 1.1.

In the reimbursement model, used in Belgium and France, consumers pay providers directly and are reimbursed by the insurer, and there is no direct relationship between the provider and insurer. By contrast, in the public contract model, used in the Netherlands and Germany, the insurer contracts directly with providers to supply specified services to consumers. Finally, in the vertically integrated model, the insurer also directly owns and manages the providers, as in the UK National Health Service prior to changes in 1990.

A further sign of the rise of the market in health care has been a move by countries with vertically integrated systems towards the public contract model: putting a 'market' structure in place by splitting the insurance/third party payer function from the provision and management of services, and making providers compete for contracts (so called 'internal 'or 'quasi-markets'). The service providers may either be publicly or privately owned or have charitable status. In countries where the public contract model already exists, the emphasis may be, not on forming but, on 're-forming' the market, with moves to strengthen third party payers and make them more proactive and effective purchasers of care on behalf of consumers. Paradoxically this may entail *integrating* the purchaser and provider functions in health maintenance organisations and other forms of 'managed care' (discussed below). In some

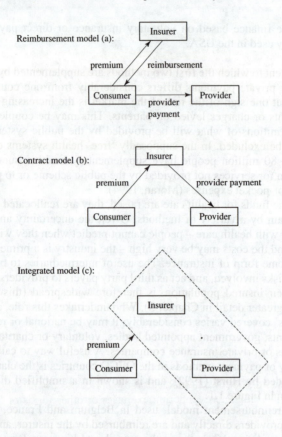

*Figure 1.1 – **Three models of paying providers by third-party payers ('insurers')***
Source: van der Ven, et al. (1994) p. 1407

cases, as in parts of Sweden, consumers have been given much greater choice of providers, who are competing for the public funds consumers are indirectly bringing with them. In other cases (the Netherlands, Germany) consumers have also been given greater choice of health insurers, who purchase health care on their behalf.

A final example of the rise of the market, alluded to by Moran (1994) is the expansion of private providers in areas where the state had a virtual monopoly in the employment of medical labour, such as Sweden, the UK and New Zealand. This is coupled with an expansion of private providers in other areas: for example contracting out or 'outsourcing' many nonclinical services to the private sector is well-established in the UK, and, increasingly, the use of private capital to build hospitals which will then be leased back to the National Health Service is replacing publicly capitalised investment.

Marketisation or privatisation?

The major focus of this book is the introduction or strengthening of market mechanisms and incentives in the health care systems of a group of advanced Western states. Are these changes to be represented as marketisation or privatisation? Freeman, in Chapter 10, argues that conceptually and analytically these are distinct phenomena, yet they are often used interchangeably because there is little agreement on what we mean by privatisation.

In analysing Conservative approaches to privatisation in the UK, Stephen Young argued in 1986 for a broad definition:

> In very broad terms privatisation can be taken to describe a set of policies which aim to limit the role of the public sector and increase the role of the private sector, while improving the performance of the remaining public sector.
>
> (Young, 1986: 236)

Young argued that it was possible to discern seven different forms of privatisation in Conservative policy:

1. Outright sales of public assets to the private sector.
2. Relaxing state monopolies (deregulation or liberalisation) by changing regulations to allow private providers to enter the market.
3. Contracting out or externalisation of services to the private sector, through competitive tendering exercises or other forms of 'market testing'.
4. Increasing private provision of services presently monopolised by public providers, which may still be publicly funded.
5. Using private investment capital to undertake development projects, for example build hospitals, the Channel Tunnel, etc.
6. Reduced subsidies and increased user charges. Consumers pay the total cost or greater proportion of the real cost of providing services.
7. Privatising from within – extending private sector practices into the public sector – imbuing the public sector with techniques 'tested developed and refined in market conditions' (Young, 1986: 243).

Although still a useful preliminary categorisation, Young's definition is too broad even for developments in the UK, let alone cross-nationally: the planned market experiments between exclusively public providers in Scandinavia were not intended to increase the opportunities for the private sector, for example.

What Young could not foresee perhaps when he wrote this article was the growing importance of initiatives which broadly fall within his

category 7 and the international pervasiveness of 'new public management' (NPM) doctrines (Hood, 1991) based on two, sometimes contradictory, streams of thought. The first is the critique of bureaucracy
represented by public choice economics which leads in the direction of
markets, competition and user choice, either through contracting out,
quasi- or internal markets, the increased involvement of private companies and not-for-profits in public service provision and capital investment (Young's categories 2, 3, 4 and 5). Secondly there has been a new
wave of managerialism based on private sector theories and practices.
This has led to a reassertion of management authority over labour, the
break-up of traditional government bureaucracies into separate more focused agencies, the extensive use of contracts or quasi-contracts to
regulate internal and external relationships, devolution of operational
autonomy down the line, the setting of clear standards and measures of
performance and a shift towards output controls rather than inputs.

Conceptually it could be argued that the new public management has
led to the *marketisation* of public services by incorporating market
methods and incentives into the management of public services in the
belief that this will improve their efficiency and effectiveness. As a consequence this may lead also to increasing *privatisation*, if for example,
more contracts are won by the private sector in tendering exercises, or
if, in the private financing of public facilities discussed above, there is a
transfer of ownership. Indeed, one of the most influential NPM texts,
Reinventing Government by Osborne and Gaebler (1992), argued that
the role of government *should* change from being largely a provider of
services delivered through state bureaucracies, and become more entrepreneurial and catalytic: governments should 'steer and not row', in
their famous phrase. Others, notably the private sector but also the voluntary and community sector, should do the rowing.[1] Marketisation and
privatisation are not interchangeable concepts therefore but, in practice,
one may lead to the other.

'Managed care' and 'managed competition'

The concepts of 'managed care' and 'managed competition' are also
central to the developments discussed in later chapters. The continual
spiral of health care inflation in the USA has led corporate business to
seek ways of reducing the bills they incur for their employees. This has
led to a move away from traditional indemnity insurance, and fee-for-
service medicine (where doctors were paid for each item of service),
since neither the provider nor the patient had any incentive to be cost-
conscious, thus driving up premiums to the employer. Instead some
form of 'managed care' now covers 75 per cent of working Americans
(Bransten, 1997). This was based originally on health maintenance organisations (HMOs) but now has a variety of forms. All are alike in
combining the insurance and delivery aspects of medical care and all

share, to varying extents, the following features:

- delivery of a comprehensive set of health services to enrollees for a prepaid premium;
- utilisation and quality controls that providers agree to accept (for example, the insurer may not sanction or pay for certain procedures, may require prior authorisation for others, require the submission of specified outcome data, etc.);
- financial incentives for patients to use the provider's facilities or designated physicians only;
- the assumption of some financial risk by doctors to make them balance patients' needs against the need for cost control.

In staff-model and group-model HMOs multispeciality groups of salaried physicians practise in facilities provided by the HMOs owners, according to agreed protocols and ways of working. The prepayment system changes the structure of incentives, and makes doctors operate in a cost-conscious fashion. In some forms of managed care physicians still work in their own offices but are signed up to different insurers, and agree to work according to their rules (independent practice organisations or IPAs). These vary in their intrusiveness and detailed control of medical practice, but as downwards pressure on costs has intensified in recent years, such controls have correspondingly intensified as well.

It should be pointed out that 'managed care' as a concept is possible in a wide variety of settings (hence the international interest in it as a means of delivering more cost-effective services), and can be accomplished with a greater degree of medical self-management. For instance, some primary care practices in the general practice fundholding scheme in the UK are piloting measures which enable them to provide or purchase comprehensive care for their enrolled patients within a global budget agreed annually with the health authority. These have many of the features of managed care but clearly operate within a very different context and health care culture.

Managed care delivered mainly through HMOs is a key component of 'managed competition' as promoted by the American economist, Alain Enthoven as the solution to the ills of the United States system for over two decades (see, for instance, Enthoven 1978, 1994; Enthoven and Kronick 1989). His ideas won astonishing acceptance as the basis for health care reform internationally, chiming well with the new pro-market political climate of the 1980s, yet with little evidence of their feasibility in the USA. The core of Enthoven's proposals for the USA is that managed care plans would compete on quality and price for insurance contracts from employers, Medicare and Medicaid and any other payers interested in low cost insurance. The competition would be regulated by public agencies who act as 'sponsors' for the consumer. They would certify approved managed care plans, define standard benefits, ensure open enrolment and monitor quality. Much is expected of the sponsor, who would be: 'an active, intelligent collective purchasing agent on the demand side ... that creates, develops, administers and enforces the rules of competition in a never-ending effort to root out market failures and to perfect the market' (Enthoven, 1994: 1416).

Costs would also be driven down by removing tax incentives for employers and individuals: only the lowest cost plans would be tax deductible. Although different forms of managed care plans (for example IPAs) would be permitted to compete, the assumption is that they would not be successful and, like traditional indemnity insurance, would be driven out of the market. Most doctors would have to be affiliated with HMOs, and most of these would be owned by insurance companies. Indeed, critics of managed competition in the USA have dubbed the proposals a form of insurance industry preservation act.[2]

When applied outside the USA, Enthoven's analysis has to take account of different institutional contexts (who should undertake the sponsor's role, for example) and different agendas. For example, Britain has managed to control its costs at the macro level very successfully, so the thrust of Enthoven's criticism of the National Health Service, written after a study visit in 1984, was directed at the effects of 'unresponsive government' and 'monopolistic professionals' to justify the incorporation of competitive incentives into the service. Marmor and Maynard (1994: 7) argue that 'this was an instance of almost pure theory being transplanted across an ocean, contextless and lacking critical evaluation as well as evidence of its efficiency', yet it was acted upon with enthusiasm, first in Britain and the Netherlands and from there travelling to Sweden, New Zealand, Australia and many other countries, a textbook case of 'lesson drawing' in public policy (Rose, 1993).

Problems of comparative analysis

The pitfalls of comparative policy analysis are now widely acknowledged (Cochrane, 1993; Hill, 1996), but avoiding them is still not easy. The first pitfall is to assume that similar terms mean the same thing in different countries, although in practice their use reflects different social meanings of which the observer from another country is unaware. Health care reform has been dominated by the language of 'markets', 'competition' and 'user choice' but a major theme of this book is the way this disguises very different concepts in varying institutional and cultural contexts. States also differ in what they regard as 'public' and 'private'. For example, Saltman and von Otter (1992) give a uniquely Swedish example of the 'private sector' when they discuss the City-Akuten ambulatory clinic in Stockholm, a successful clinic in the city centre providing convenient and accessible services for office workers on a walk-in basis. The clinic is funded by the county council out of its funds for ambulatory care. Patients pay the same small fee they would pay in a 'public' primary health centre. The physicians who work there are salaried public employees, working in their off-duty and vacation hours. This can accumulate to four months a year, following a county council decision in the late 1970s to compensate them with time off rather than salary increments. Hence:

> Despite its formal status as a 'private' firm ... the success of the City-Akuten clinic directly reflects the fact it serves predominantly public sector patients and operates almost entirely with public sector resources; it is staffed by public employees, utilizing public-sector-created off-duty time, and is paid with publicly collected and distributed funds.
>
> (Saltman and von Otter, 1992: 45)

Given such complexities, the first reaction is to give up comparative analysis altogether on the basis that all cultures are unique, but the value of escaping parochialism no longer makes that an option. 'Social scientific teeth are gritted, problems acknowledged and comparisons made' (Cochrane 1993: 6) but, as Cochrane points out, the legacy of these fears survives and may give rise to a collection of individual case studies which are only tenuously linked together.

> A great deal of supposedly comparative work looks rather too much like an unconnected series of chapters (usually written by national experts) each summarizing the experience of one country and expecting the reader to draw his or her own conclusions.
>
> (Cochrane, 1993: 6)

The alternative approach is to move towards aggregated statistical data, compiled by international agencies like the United Nations or OECD, which makes it possible to compare features such as levels of public spending on particular social programmes, patterns of income distribution, employment, health status indicators and so on. It then becomes possible to formulate and test hypotheses on what might have contributed to these differences, and construct typologies using different combinations of variables (see, for instance, Castles, 1982; Esping-Andersen, 1985; Heidenheimer *et al.*, 1990). But not only is the data used for comparison sometimes suspect, once again reflecting individual state differences in definitions and data collection systems, aggregate analysis also leaves huge explanatory gaps as to why and how observed differences and correlations have occurred over time. Once again we have to return to the case study for explanations.

As far as current health sector reform strategies are concerned, the case for detailed description and analysis by 'national experts' is strong. The reforms are still comparatively recent and there is a good deal of ignorance and misapprehension about outcomes and effects. Yet at the same time promarket, procompetitive recipes for reforming health care (often as part of a wider package of public management reforms) are being vigorously marketed by bodies like the World Bank or International Monetary Fund in Central and Eastern Europe and the developing world (sometimes the receipt of aid is conditional on accepting such solutions), and by international accountancy and management consultants like Anderson Consultants, Coopers and Lybrand or KMPG Peat Marwick who operate at a global level (James and Manning, 1996).

We have attempted to deal with the problems outlined by Cochrane above, first by setting the case studies within a detailed exploration of the global context within which health care restructuring has taken place, which is often neglected or given passing mention in some other studies (see, for instance, Ham, 1997). Paradoxically, as Cochrane observes, this makes it easier to identify and explain the reasons for individual differences when they do occur. Secondly, we have made our enquiry question-led rather than data-driven, and thirdly we have focused on a set of countries which are broadly comparable on the following dimensions:

- all fall within the category of mature Western capitalist democracies;
- all fall within the OECD 'core' group of public management reformers, with the exception of Germany (James and Manning, 1996).

The following section explains the rationale for these countries' inclusion in greater detail and outlines the contents and scope of each chapter.

Contents and scope

After the introductory chapter the book begins with a global overview by Michael Moran, setting out the political and economic context in which health care reform became more pressing in Western democracies in the 1980s and the reasons why government elites looked more favourably at procompetitive solutions. Moran's key argument is that health care systems in capitalist liberal democracies are embedded in market economies which are increasingly interdependent on a *global* scale, but operate within *national* systems of democratic politics. In addition, they:

> … are themselves significant concentrations of economic might and political pressure. They are not simply subsystems responding to wider capitalist or democratic environments. As concentrations of economic activity, complex organisations and constellations of political influence they are major influences on that environment.
>
> (Chapter 2: 20)

From this central thesis Moran unravels the tensions and contradictions which follow from the twin face of health care – as a core institution of welfare and as a collection of industries which may be of critical importance in national strategies of competitiveness in the global economy.

A notable feature of health care debates in the 1980s and 1990s is the extent to which issues and problems have been framed by the discourse of economics, as a result of the remarkable rise in influence and numbers of health economists. As Moran pointed out in an earlier paper (1994) the fact that the United States health care debate is about costs and efficiency (rather than equity and access) is in no small measure due to the ability of health economists to penetrate the relevant policy networks: for example, health economists dominate the Health Care Financing Administration, the federal agency set up to administer the publicly financed programmes of Medicare and Medicaid. In this role the agency is also the most important source of data and analysis about the US health care 'crisis' at federal level. From this platform promarket American health economists have been influential on a world stage, through (for example) American dominance of international bodies like the World Bank.

John Appleby's chapter serves the important function, therefore, of outlining what economists mean by efficient markets, why markets fail and the extent to which health care – as an economic commodity – meets the conditions necessary for an efficient market to operate. From there it examines different responses to perceived failures in both market and nonmarket systems, arguing that policy makers have tried to play a complex game, utilising specific market tools or instruments to deal with particular problems (in particular improving technical efficiency) in what may still remain largely publicly funded and/or provided systems. Finally, Appleby explores some of the issues that have arisen in applying market tools in health care, both on the supply and demand sides, and in relation to the regulation of the whole system.

The individual case studies start with the USA, as the source of promarket ideas in health care. In Chapter 3, Ted Marmor traces the growth of pro-competitive ideas in American medical politics from the 1970s onwards. Marmor points out that the ingenuity of promarket health economists in devising ways of 'managing' competition to deal with the real world of imperfect health care markets created the need for extensive and detailed state regulation, an ironical outcome given the anti-government bias of their endeavours. In practice, and as Appleby also points out, regulation is a tricky business, often leading to perverse incentives and unintended outcomes, because in health care the regulated know more about their business than the regulators and are usually in a good position to outwit them.

Marmor goes on to analyse in depth President Clinton's ill-fated attempt at comprehensive health care reform, which collapsed in 1994, the reasons why he failed and developments thereafter, developments which may be significant for the rest of the world and in particular for the USA's neighbour, Canada.

One reason for including Canada in the countries selected for examination is its influence on internal US debates, both as a role model for those who advocate a 'single payer'[3] model of financing health care and for those who wish to protect the status quo. Canada's system of universal public coverage for health care was only completed in the early 1970s. Before then, when its funding system was more similar to that in the USA, health care costs consumed a share of national income that was virtually identical in both countries. What was striking to American audiences (but would not surprise Europeans) was the fact that Canada achieved universal coverage with lower expenditures on health care. In 1971 expenditure as a proportion of GDP was 7.4 per cent in Canada and 7.5 per cent in the USA. By 1987 Canada's proportion was 8.9 per cent whilst growth in the USA had continued exorably upwards to 11.3 per cent, and by 1993 the figures had reached 10.2 per cent and 14.1 per cent respectively. (Figure 1.2 shows the growth in total health spending as a proportion of Gross Domestic Product for the seven countries discussed in the book; Table 1.1 shows the proportion of public expenditure in 1993.)

*Table 1.1   **Public expenditure on health as a proportion of total expenditure, 1993***

Variables	USA	Canada	UK	New Zealand	Netherlands	Sweden	Germany
-Pub. Exp. on Health /Total Health Exp.(%)	43.9	71.9	83.0	77.2	77.7	82.9	70.2

Source: OECD health data (credes/OECD)

Advocates of the Canadian system in the USA showed that savings in administration and insurance overheads were the main reasons for the lower costs in Canada (Himmelstein and Woolhandler, 1986). On some estimates these account for half the total cost difference between the two systems (Evans *et al.*, 1989), and include the costs of determining coverage, eligibility and risk status; marketing expenses; providers' accounting costs in complying with the documentation requirements of multiple insurers; direct paying and billing procedures to patients, as well as shareholders' profits. Even the US General Accounting Office estimates that the USA could achieve universal coverage without extra cost if it could match the level of administrative costs achieved by Canada (see Chapter 5).

Ranged against these views are the weight of corporate interests, in particular the private insurance companies who have every incentive to depict a different scene: disaffected doctors, waiting lists for treatment and restrictions on consumer choice (for detailed rebuttals see Deber, 1993; Evans *et al.*, 1989; Himmelstein and Woolhandler, 1992). Deber and Baranek's chapter in this book shows how both sides of the argument have sometimes taken a one-sided view or misrepresented the real problems Canada faces today. Canada's system has been a success story and a source of pride to its citizens but today is under great strain from the effects of severe economic and fiscal pressures which have become entwined with Canada's constitutional crisis.

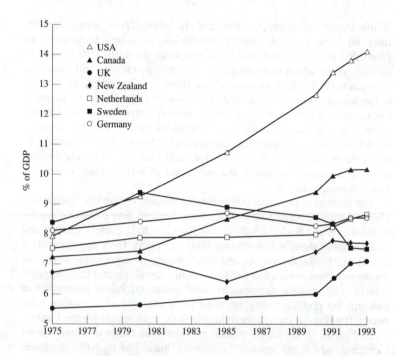

Source: OECD health data (credes/OECD) version #3.6 (1995)

Figure 1.2 **Total expenditure on health as a % of GDP – 1970-1993.**

Deber and Baranek point out that 35 per cent of total revenue collected by federal government had to be paid as interest on the national debt in 1996, and provincial governments are beginning to fall into similar straits as a consequence of years of deficit financing. As both federal and provincial government face up to the spending cuts necessary to balance budgets again, Deber and Baranek chart the effects of this on what still remains the world's second most expensive health care system, and conclude that under these economic and political pressures Canada is introducing markets at the margin – albeit substantial margins like long-term care – and privatising by attrition and default.

The next chapters (6 to 9) look at four countries at the forefront of health care reform which has been closely intertwined with their early and widespread adoption of NPM: the UK, New Zealand, the Netherlands, and Sweden. James and Manning (1996) argue that these four, together with Australia, Canada and the USA form the core OECD group of public management reformers about which most has been written, although the doctrines and techniques of NPM have spread much more widely throughout the OECD and beyond. In health care reform the Netherlands adopted a framework of 'managed competition' in the Dekker report in 1988, closely followed by the UK in the government

White Paper 'Working for Patients' in 1989. These ideas then influenced New Zealand, already undertaking a radical programme of promarket economic and social reforms since the early 1980s, with an official report which recommended similar wide-ranging and sweeping changes to the health care system. Finally in Sweden, where health care is the administrative responsibility of county councils, some councils began to experiment with 'planned market' experiments of various kinds, the best known being the 'Stockholm model' and the 'Dalarna model'. However, though the language of reform was very similar in the different countries, it was transplanted into very different institutional and cultural contexts: the substance of reform rapidly took on new guises and directions.

The authors of these chapters (Wendy Ranade for the UK, Jacqueline Cumming and George Salmond for New Zealand, Ray Robinson for the Netherlands and Richard Saltman for Sweden) have closely tracked and written about these reforms since their inception. Here they provide a detailed analysis of progress and their varying fortunes in the course of implementation, which has produced some surprising and unanticipated effects. The authors examine to what extent reformers succeeded in tackling the problems they intended to tackle, and whether they have been left with new ones, concluding with their prognosis for the future.

In Chapter 9, Richard Freeman examines the rather unusual case of Germany, which has remained relatively untouched by NPM doctrines and promarket recipes for health care reform. Yet here too policy makers experience similar problems of efficiency and cost, and have belatedly learnt to speak the language of competition and consumer choice. Price competition has been introduced between pharmaceutical producers, and more recently the sickness funds (insurers) have been allowed to compete for enrollees. Competition in this instance, however, has taken a strange form since state regulation – of prices, benefit packages, calculation of insurance premiums, and so on – is tighter than ever, and there is little left on which to compete. From his analysis of the German health sector, Freeman concludes that such an outcome is only understandable in terms of the structural features of the system, previous historic conflicts in the health sector, and federal government's continuing search for control.

Finally, Chapter 11 tries to summarise the complexity of our data, and returns to the questions posed at the beginning: what were the common pressures or triggers for health care reform and what explains the emergence of the new market orthodoxy as a policy response? How were market mechanisms selectively applied in different states and with what objectives in mind? What are the effects (both intentional and unintentional) of the market experiment in health care, and, as some states try now to take a different direction, what kind of legacy has been bequeathed?

Notes

1. James and Manning (1996) note that one effect of the spread of NPM internationally, and particularly the extensive contracting out of services to the private sector, has been the growth of large specialist suppliers who may tender for contracts in several countries.
2. Enthoven has propounded his theories in the USA through the Jackson Hole group which he founded with Dr Paul Ellwood, considered to be the father of HMOs and now the director of a health policy research institute, Interstudy. The group comprises academics, representatives from the largest health insurers, pharmaceutical and hospital industries and some large corporations who meet informally at Jackson Hole, Dr Ellwood's vacation home.
3. The single payer option in the USA would have replaced the present system of employer coverage, private insurance, Medicaid and Medicare by creating a single public system of health insurance financed through payroll and income taxes. The 'single payer' in question refers to one health insurer who collects contributions and pays providers, and this could be state governments or federal government. In Canada this role is performed by provincial governments who administer health insurance plans which must comply with federal guidelines in order to receive federal resources.

References

Bransten, L. (1997) 'The Americas: US health care costs', *Financial Times*, 25 March: 8.

Castles, F. (1982) *The Impact of Parties: Politics and Policies in Democratic Capitalist States*, London: Sage.

Cochrane, A. (1993) 'Comparative approaches and social policy', in A. Cochrane and J. Clarke (eds) *Comparing Welfare States: Britain in International Context*, London: Sage/Open University Press.

Deber, R. B.(1993) 'Canadian Medicare: Can it work in the United States? Will it survive in Canada?', *American Journal of Law and Medicine,* **19** (1 and 2): 75–93.

Enthoven, A. C. (1978) 'Consumer choice health plan: A national health insurance proposal based on regulated competition in the private sector', *New England Journal of Medicine (*23 and 30 March): 650–58 and 709–20.

Enthoven, A.C. (1994) 'On the ideal market structure for third-party purchasing of health care', *Social Science and Medicine*, **39** (10): 1413–24.

Enthoven, A. C. and Kronick, R. (1989) 'A consumer choice health plan for the 1990s', *New England Journal of Medicine*, **320** (1 and 2): 29–37 and 94–101.

Esping-Andersen, G. (1985) *Politics Against Markets: The Social Democratic Road to Power*, Princeton, New Jersey: Princeton University Press.

Evans, R. G. *et al.* (1989) 'Controlling health expenditures: The Canadian reality', *New England Journal of Medicine*, **120**(9): 571–7.

Ham, C. (ed.) (1997) *Health Care Reform*, Buckingham: Open University Press.

Heidenheimer, A. J., Heclo, H. and Adams, C.T. (1990) *Comparative Public Policy: The Politics of Social Choice in America, Europe and Japan* (3rd edn), New York: St Martins Press.

Hill, M. (1996) *Social Policy: A Comparative Analysis*, Hemel Hempstead: Prentice Hall and Harvester Wheatsheaf.

Himmelstein, D. and Woolhandler, S. (1986) 'Cost without benefit: Administrative waste in US health care', *New England Journal of Medicine*, **314**: 441–5.

Himmelstein, D. and Woolhandler, S. (1992) *The National Health Program Chartbook*, Monroe, Maine: Common Courage Press.

Hood, C. (1991) 'A public management for all seasons?', *Public Administration*, **69**: 3–19.

Hurst, J. (1992) *The Reform of Health Care: A Comparative Analysis of Seven OECD Countries*, Paris: OECD.

James, O. and Manning, N. (1996) 'Public management reform: A global perspective', *Politics*, **16**(3): 143–9.

Marmor, T.R. (1995) *The Politics of Medical Care Reform in Mature Welfare States: Fact, Fiction, and Faction*. Paper given to Four Country Conference on Health Care Reform and Health Care Policies in the United States, Canada, Germany and the Netherlands, Rotterdam, 23–25 February.

Marmor, T. R. and Maynard, A. (1994) 'Cross-national transfer of health policy ideas: The case of "managed competition". Paper prepared for panel of Comparative Health Policy Study Group, International Political Studies Association, Berlin 21–25 August.

Moran, M. (1994) 'Reshaping the health care state', *Government and Opposition*, **19**(1): 48–64.

Newhouse, J. (1996) 'Health reform in the United States', *The Economic Journal*, **106**: 1713–24.

Osborne, R. and Gaebler, T. (1992) *Reinventing Government*, Wokingham: Addison Wesley.

Rose, R. (1993) *Lesson-drawing in Public Policy*, Chatham, New Jersey: Chatham House.

van der Ven, W., Schut, F. T and Rutten, F.H.(1994) 'Forming and reforming the market for third-party purchasing of health care', *Social Science and Medicine*, **39** (10): 1405–12.

Salter, B. (1995) 'The private sector and the NHS: Redefining the welfare state', *Policy and Politics*, **23**(1): 17–30.

Saltman, R. and von Otter, C. (1992) *Planned Markets and Public Competition*, Buckingham: Open University Press.

Young, S. (1986) 'The nature of privatisation in Britain 1979–1985', *West European Politics*, **9**: 235–52.

CHAPTER 2

Explaining the rise of the market in health care

MICHAEL MORAN

Two temptations in the study of health care policy

The recent history of health care in the advanced industrial world is puzzling. The puzzle is: why has so much reform been influenced by market ideologies?

Posing this puzzle presents another: what does 'market' mean? It is notoriously the case that it can signify different things. Indeed it is precisely this quality that confers rhetorical power. A formula such as 'managed market' – like its big sister, market socialism – offers a reconciliation of two social forms usually thought to be in Manichean opposition. My solution to the problem of definition is crude. A market can mean many things, but one thing it certainly means is summed up by Maynard: 'a network of buyers (purchasers) and sellers (providers) who exchange money and services' (1995: 51). The spread of the market in recent years involves the spread of these kinds of networks. Our puzzle can now be more precisely expressed: why is the buying and selling of health care goods and services increasingly common, and why is there such urging for it to become commoner still?

Answering this question presents us with two temptations, both of which should be resisted: one is to explain the change purely in the language of economic imperatives; the other to explain it purely in the language of political ideology.

An explanation in the language of economic imperatives fastens onto the problem of cost containment. With the important exception of the United States, health care policy across the advanced capitalist world showed a distinctive pattern in the 30 years after the end of the Second World War. The proceeds of the 'long boom' in the 30 glorious years after the close of the war helped fund a great expansion in welfare entitlements. States that initially led in guaranteeing free, or nearly free, health care for some citizens moved to complete universalism, and 'laggards' caught up, especially after 1960. The consequence is well known, and is encapsulated in the data set accumulated by the OECD: across the OECD nations by the 1970s, with the exception of the United States, the percentage of national populations with entitlements to free or nearly free health care approached one hundred (see, for instance, OECD, 1987: 54–9).

Since the middle of the 1970s, policy makers have been trying to cope with the aftermath of that expansion. The end of the 'long boom' put paid to the economic machine which created the resources for universalism; and universalism itself established health care systems where demand, unconstrained by a budgetary limit, was potentially infinite. By this account, then, the history of health care policy for the last two decades is a history of the search for cost containment, and the resort to market mechanisms is an attempt to impose limits on the unconstrained demands for care from citizens.

This explanation is unsatisfactory for three reasons. First, it flies in the face of evidence that universalism has not been incompatible with cost containment. It is true that the expansion of entitlements was accompanied by a rise in health care spending; but the remarkable feature of the 1980s was that states that had completed the march to universalism were strikingly successful in containing costs. Cost containment, of course, included some market mechanisms, like cost sharing, but only as part of a range of instruments, of which global budgets seem to have been the most effective. (For the supporting evidence see OECD, 1992). Despite the success of cost containment, the pressure to shift to market systems of resource raising and allocation did not diminish.

These observations are connected to a second reason for scepticism. It is well known that, although all OECD health care systems experienced a long-term rise in the resources allocated to health care, there were substantial differences in the pace of spending growth. We might expect, therefore, that the introduction of market 'disciplines' would be greatest in the most heavily burdened systems, and least in those systems where costs were already contained. This is not so. The most obvious confounding instance is the United Kingdom: it combined universalism with successful cost containment, but was nevertheless a leader in experiments with new market mechanisms. Indeed the British experience suggests even more perverse connections, for there is some, admittedly not decisive, evidence that since the reforms introduced from the early 1990s the record of cost containment has been less impressive than hitherto (see Moran, 1995). If the resort to the market is a response to problems of cost containment created by universalism there must be a substantial rationality deficit in the policy process in health care.

The third difficulty with the notion that the turn to the market is the result of the search for cost containment concerns the origin of ideologies of market allocation. Their rise is in part the product of the international diffusion of ideas, with the United State as source. The policy history of recent years amounts to 'Americanisation'. Theories of planned markets, for instance, emerged out of policy debates created by the chaos of the American health care system. Three decades ago the United States was a 'laggard' looking to Europe for reform inspiration; in the 1990s the traffic has been in the other direction, as the dazzling career of Alain Enthoven illustrates. Yet if market reform is viewed as an effort at cost containment this is an odd state of affairs, since the

American system is notoriously the most ineffective at containing costs. Taking lessons in health care policy from the United States is like receiving instruction in seamanship from the crew of the *Titanic*.

Of course there is more to 'cost containment' than curbing the global total of resources allocated to health care. The great rise in levels of health care spending, even in parsimonious systems like the United Kingdom, inevitably focused attention on other aspects of costs: on the way the burden of paying for care fell on different groups; on the hypothesised connection between particular methods of paying for care and the micro-efficiency in the resource allocation process; on the link between methods of raising and allocating resources and the sensitivity with which health care institutions dealt with patients. Saltman and von Otter (1992) have offered an explanation for the widespread experimentation with markets in the United Kingdom and Scandinavia which does make a realistic connection with problems of resource raising and allocation. They argue that such systems were effectively 'command-like': that is, they raised and distributed resources by administrative command (for instance by levying taxes) rather than through market mechanisms. They suffered from many of the known problems of command economies, inefficiencies and insensitivity to consumer demand. Market experimentation is an attempt in these systems to cope with those problems.

This account, though appealing, is insufficient. The rise of the market is not confined to the 'command-like' systems of Scandinavia and the United Kingdom, so we need an explanation that will transcend these nations. Saltman and von Otter nevertheless give a clue as to what that explanation might be. The realism of their account lies in its recognition that the rise of the market, like the rise of any other social order, is produced by strategic decisions made by powerful interests. Its rise is not a simple response to cost burdens, but is determined by the strategic calculations of those interests and the success with which calculations shape policy outcomes. Those calculations, in turn, are mediated by ideologies: structures of ideas that emerge and prosper because they can legitimise the interests of powerful groups.

But these insights lead to the second temptation which needs to be resisted: the temptation to reduce the rise of the market to a case of pure ideology. A parsimonious account of the rise of the market in health care can link its ascendancy to the ideological crisis of the wider welfare state, and even to the wider crisis of social democratic ideology. Though there is considerable dispute about both the meaning of these 'crises', and about the evidence for their existence (Alber, 1988), there is no doubt that the rise of market ideologies in health care did indeed have some connection with a diminished confidence on the part of many governing elites in the capacity of an interventionist state to guarantee social citizenship. But the rise of the market in health care cannot be 'read off' from the wider difficulties of the welfare state or of social democracy. Trying to do so simply flies in the face of the evidence accumulated by the country case studies in this volume: that the form and penetration of market ideologies depends heavily on the particular national setting, and not on some universal *Zeitgeist*. Ideology is important, but that importance is mediated through particular national settings, and shaped by the calculations of powerful interests.

Allowing ideology primacy also incurs the fallacy of treating health care systems as mere subsystems of the welfare state. Confronting that fallacy allows us to formulate an account of health care politics which avoids the twin temptations of reducing change to a matter of either economic imperatives or ideological constructions. The best way to express this wider understanding of the forces shaping health care policy is to recognise something shared by the health care systems of advanced industrial countries: they are embedded in particular kinds of economic and political institutions.

The embedded nature of health care institutions

Examine the national health care systems selected for case study in this volume, or the larger group (the OECD nations) usually analysed comparatively. They share three features. First, they operate within market economies in an interdependent world. Second, they operate within national systems of democratic politics. A summary of these two characteristics is that health care systems are embedded within capitalist democracies. Third, health care systems are themselves significant concentrations of economic might and political pressure. They are not simply subsystems responding to wider capitalist or democratic environments. As concentrations of economic activity, complex organisations and constellations of political influence they are major influences on that environment.

Consider first the case of economic embeddedness. Viewed thus, health care systems are part of industrial politics. Health care is a personal service, but it is a personal service delivered in large economic organisations using the products, in many cases, of advanced manufacturing technology. High technology plays a vital part in modern health care, notably through pharmaceuticals and much medical equipment. The fate of these high technology health care industries is vital to the success of any capitalist economy. That importance can be measured in many ways: by the sheer size of the manufacturing industries involved in the production of health care goods; by the strategic importance of these industries in renewing and extending the technological base of advanced capitalist economies; by the way the economic actors in these industries – who include some of the biggest multinational firms in the world economy – compete for market share and profits. In the advanced capitalist world – and especially in the G7 countries – states are intimately involved in the competition between these firms. Beyond high technology, health care institutions are also large industrial undertak-

ings vital to local and regional economies: consider only the employment impact of large hospitals in the cities of the advanced industrial
world, and the way that employment impact complicates hospital planning.

The industrial politics of health care are shaped by competition on an
international scale. The democratic politics of health care are also competitive, but competition is largely within nations. Democracy institu-
tionalises political competition: some is between parties for votes; some
is between organised interests within and outside health care systems.
As in other parts of the welfare state, the delivery of health care is done
through powerful occupations. The way organised interests operate is in
part a function of the way wider democratic arrangements work – and
as significant organised interests, health care institutions themselves
contribute to the way democratic politics function.

In short: health care systems help shape capitalist economies and are
shaped by those economies; they help shape democratic politics, and
are shaped by democracy. This simple insight provides a clue to the rise
of the market in health care. Health care systems share the common feature of embeddedness in the institutions of democratic capitalism. The
rise of the market, a common experience across health care systems,
must be traceable to some common developments in the way health
care systems are embedded in democratic capitalism. We can explore
these changes in the two spheres of industrial politics and democratic
politics.

Industrial politics and the politics of health care

That health care politics are partly industrial politics has two implications: the intersection between the health care system and the wider
economy critically shapes health care policy; and the changing character of industrial politics helps explain the turn to the market. I illustrate
using examples from two levels: from the level of national economic systems; and from the level of a sector, the medical technology industries.

The search for competitive efficiency in national economies has intimately shaped health care policy. The history of expansion before the
middle of the 1970s left health care systems in absolute terms very large
indeed: health became the 'world's biggest industry', in the words of
Jencks and Schieber (1991: 1). This sheer size means that any *general*
pressures to cut costs in the search for efficiency are bound to involve
health care. Since the end of the 'long boom', all capitalist economies
have been under precisely that sort of pressure. The pressure to ensure
competitive advantage is intense. National economies have become increasingly meshed together. Success or failure depends utterly on maintaining competitive advantage, and maintaining that advantage has been
seen as partly a matter of cutting costs. Containing costs – at which
health care institutions have turned out to be quite effective – is neither

here nor there in this sort of world. Policy is driven, not primarily by what happens inside health care institutions, but by the wider context of economic policy. Since no national economy can insulate itself from wider global forces, the fate of health care policy is heavily influenced by how the national economy copes with these global forces.

These observations help explain why the success of health care systems in containing costs in the 1980s nevertheless failed to still the demands for market reforms: the issue was not the success of health care cost containment alone but the contribution the health care economy could make to the struggle for national economic competitiveness. Three different cases illustrate this point: they correspond to cases of economic crisis, economic interdependence and hegemonic decline.

First, some nations have radically changed institutions or entitlements as a direct result of a more general national effort to cope with economic failure. In their different ways the radical British and New Zealand changes are the product of such forces. The British reforms originated in the Thatcherite efforts to reverse the decline of the British economy. The Thatcher revolution was designed to do this by reconstructing public institutions and citizen entitlements. The object was to shrink the role of the state and to displace welfare entitlements based on social citizenship with claims dependent on contracts bought in markets. The historical success of the old NHS in containing global costs was an irrelevance in these revolutionary circumstances. Indeed, the surprising feature of the British reforms is not their radical nature but their modesty. In health care there has not yet been a great abolition of the entitlements of social citizenship, nor a wholesale dismantling of the public institutions of health care. That surprising lack of radicalism is connected to the democratic political circumstances in which policy has to be made: as Chapter 6 demonstrates there have been a number of occasions, notably in 1983, when the government was forced by fear of the electorate to step back from radical change. New Zealand's reforms were also part of a wider attempt to restructure the welfare state in the face of the economic difficulties caused by the loss of the country's European markets for its agricultural products and, like the British reforms, the radical character dictated by economics has been partly compromised by the pressure of competitive democratic politics. (On the connection between the New Zealand reforms and the wider problems of welfare citizenship see the collection edited by Sharp, 1994).

One group of nations is struggling to cope with economic crisis. A second is locked into arrangements that magnify interdependence. The countries that entered and (unlike the UK) stayed in the European Monetary System are the obvious example. Ferrera (1995) has charted how the growing limitations on health care entitlements in Italy since the end of the 1970s grew out of policy restrictions created by membership of the EMS, and particularly by the belief of governing elites that membership of the system restricted the monetary and fiscal policies which any member state could independently pursue. The same impulses lie behind the attacks on entitlements in France and Germany designed to ensure that these national economies meet the Maastricht criteria for entry into European Monetary Union. Once again the point is not the success or otherwise of health care institutions as agents of global cost containment or micro-efficiency. Ideology has shaped a wider set of policy goals (for instance, 'convergence' as in the Maastricht criteria) which dictate the terms of health care reform.

The final case – policy prompted by hegemonic decline – concerns the United States, the one country which has conspicuously failed to implement any sort of effective cost containment. The rise of health care reform to the top of the American political agenda is not due only to this failure; it is due to the way the failure of cost containment has meshed with debates about American economic decline, especially in the face of Japanese competition. The American system of health insurance places much of the burden of increasing costs on large industrial employers who had bargained generous health insurance arrangements with employees. The penetration of American markets for products like automobiles by Japanese firms has convinced sections of the American economic elite that part of American uncompetitiveness lies in the high cost of care and in the way much of that cost is shouldered by large industrial firms. (For the structural factors linking insurance costs to competitiveness see Chollet, 1994.)

The American case emphasises the importance of something that at present is poorly understood: the role of ideology in mediating policy responses to the pressures of international competition. The arguments between professional economists show that the hypothesised connection between generous health insurance arrangements in the workplace and the competitiveness of American firms against Japanese rivals is dubious (see Reinhardt, 1989). The key point, however, is not the scientific truth or otherwise of the hypothesised connection between high health insurance costs and industrial competitiveness; it is the way this hypothesised connection can be invoked by competing interests struggling to fashion an American response to the Japanese industrial challenge. In precisely the same fashion, it matters little whether a radical reform of the NHS could help halt British economic decline; it matters a great deal that the ideology which has dominated the debate about how to reverse decline suggests that this is precisely what is needed. (Half a century ago prevailing ideologies of national planning helped legitimise the National Health Service at foundation; in the 1980s and 1990s prevailing ideologies helped delegitimise the 'command' system established in 1948.) We presently have little understanding of how ideologies of market competition spread internationally, and how they are carried into particular policy subsystems like that concerned with health care. Examples from other arenas – like the spread internationally of the idea of privatisation – suggest that policy entrepreneurs, management consultants with a potential financial interest in managing the reform process, and institutions like the World Bank that assume a 'global' policy role, may all be important, but we lack a good case study of this process in the health field. (For the views of the World Bank on health service reform see World Bank, 1993.) I have emphasised how the search for national efficiency shapes health care policy because the examples illustrate how the ideologies that prevail in debates about national economic choices can be appropriated by strategic actors within the narrower health care field itself. To leave the discussion there would, however, suggest that health care policy is only responding to larger external forces. The industrial politics of health care amounts to more: health care institutions are major economic actors in their own right; they have an internal dynamic which itself shapes the sort of reform choices that can be made; and the case of medical technology demonstrates these points.

The medical technology sector encompasses a wide span of industries and products: it ranges from products created by advanced laboratory science (for example, many pharmaceutical products and diagnostic imaging devices like body scanners) to mass produced, technologically simple devices (for example swabs and syringes). This heterogeneous collection is united by one important feature: states played a key part in creating the modern medical technology industries. States funded the research base, shaped the markets and regulated those markets. One reason for the critical historical role of states was war. Before the Second World War the industries were technologically simple. In the intervening period they have been transformed. In pharmaceuticals, for instance, the 'therapeutic revolution' associated with the discovery of sulphanilamide penicillin initiated, in Temin's words, 'a revolution in the production and distribution of medical drugs.' (Temin, 1980: 58). Before that revolution, drug companies manufactured a limited range of products dictated by a fixed technology, and engaged in no large-scale research; after it, they became leaders in R&D, the range of products widened greatly, and success in innovation became a key to success in markets. The military commitments of the state also transformed parts of the medical devices industry. For instance, sonar technology, which is the root of modern diagnostic imaging, was developed to hunt down the enemy in the Second World War.

Nor was this a once and for all affair. The continuing search for business by firms in the military equipment industry meant that some of the most significant innovations in diagnostic imaging came from adaptations by these firms, seeking new business as traditional defence markets contracted. IBM, General Electric, McDonnell Douglas, all major defence contractors, are also leading health technology contractors. The route originally opened by war cleared the way for a sustained link between high technology innovation and medical innovation. The most important connection is between the micro-electronic revolution and medical devices innovation. Micro-circuitry and advances in the storing and digitalisation of information have been at the root of many of the greatest advances, notably in 'big ticket' technology such as scanners.

Some sense of the historical break is communicated by Trajtenberg in his study of the adoption and diffusion of CT scanners:

> there is a key commonality to the great majority of items now figuring in the available menu of goods, namely the ever growing power of electronics. In fact, there is probably as much in common today between, say, a jet fighter and a CT scanner, as between either of them and its corresponding predecessor of a generation ago.
>
> (Trajtenberg, 1990: 2)

Much of the technologically dynamic part of the medical goods industries is a legacy of the great military conflicts between states in the middle decades of the twentieth century. As Foote summarily puts it: 'The [second world] war affected innovation in dramatic ways. At the discovery stage, medical device innovation was stimulated and encouraged. Many technological innovations in materials science, radar, ultrasound, and other advancements had significant medical implications in the postwar period' (Foote, 1992: 52). That technological dynamism has been maintained by the involvement of the state in the postwar years. After the Second World War, states took over the role of promoting basic research and development. The state's role also went beyond laying the knowledge base. It shaped markets, notably through regulation, and created markets through its purchasing power.

The medical goods industries prospered by applying technologies originally created through state competition in arenas other than health care, like war. The chance to exploit these opportunities was created by the historical alliance of scientific medicine and industrial capitalism. That alliance in turn was supported by the cultural authority of science and technology, by its demonstrable claims to therapeutic effectiveness when applied to health care. The result was to create a Schumpetrian health care economy, where competitive advantage turned on successful innovation: in the medical technology industries R&D, not cost control, has been the key to success in markets. In supporting this vast R&D effort, states created industries whose success was in turn vital to the wider economy.

Three examples from different jurisdictions make the point. Consider first diagnostic imaging technologies and the American economy. For much of the 1970s and 1980s the American diagnostic imaging market was growing at around 8 per cent per annum, a rate comparable to that achieved in high technology sectors like computing (Trajtenberg, 1990: 45–9). There were thus powerful forces encouraging the creation of a market for glamorous and expensive pieces of diagnostic imaging equipment. Patient safety, therapeutic efficacy or cost effectiveness could not command policy. Here is Banta on the diffusion of CT scanners:

> Despite more than five years of experience with CT scanning, its

usefulness and ultimate place in medical care are largely unknown. The development and diffusion of CT scanners took place without formal and detailed proof of their safety and efficacy.

(Banta, 1980: 263)

The second example is British. The British economy has had few outstanding successes for a century. One exception is pharmaceuticals, where British firms remain in the global first rank. The promotion of continued British pharmaceutical success is vital to a state with a declining economy and few other world beating firms. Finally, consider the dramatic impact which success in the world medical technology markets can have on a small state and economy. Denmark, with only 0.1 per cent of world population, has nearly 4 per cent of the world's export market in medicaments, and nearly 5 per cent of the market in orthopaedic appliances:

Over the past forty years, Danish industries supplying the health sector have experienced remarkable development and have become a large industrial sector, both in comparison with the rest of Danish manufacturing industry and with the world market for health care products.

(Lotz, 1993: 175)

Denmark has over 20 per cent of the world market in hearing aids. That extraordinary domination has its origins in public policy: 'The remarkable success of the Danish hearing aid producers stems from three sources: audiological research, audiological service, and public procurement policy' (Lotz, 1993: 177).

These three examples are designed to show that by the time cost containment became a pressing problem in health care, states had helped create technologically innovative medical goods industries, whose very success made them vital to wider national prosperity. The size and technological sophistication of the medical goods industries presented policy makers with a dilemma: they had simultaneously to try to curb technological innovation (in the interests of suppressing demand for health care) and to promote technological innovation (in the interests of fostering national industrial success). The resolution of this dilemma leads to market-based health care reform. National industrial strategy ruled out suppressing the supply of innovation from the industries. The alternative was to turn to market mechanisms (cost sharing with consumers, squeezing more efficiency out of service providers by competition) in order to push down consumer demand.

The medical goods industries are a striking illustration of how embeddedness in the market economy shapes health care policy. But the story told above also contains another skein. In trying to manage the consequences of successful technological innovation in health care, states are attempting to manage forces in two different geographical spheres: one sphere is the global, where markets are organised; the other is the national, where health care systems are organised. The most rational strategy for a state, but one that is virtually impossible to pursue, is to promote successful technological innovation in its medical goods industries, but to export all the results of that innovation. The tension between what world markets demand and what institutions organised on a national scale demand is highlighted when we turn to the second kind of embeddedness: in the world of democratic politics.

Democratic politics and the politics of health care

The health care systems that developed in the advanced capitalist world after the Second World War were, in general, in democracies, but they were democracies where health care politics was insulated from democratic forces. The insulation was encapsulated in one of the most authoritative and influential accounts of the health care political arena offered in the postwar years, that by Alford (1975), identifying patients as a repressed interest in health care systems.

That repression was due to three factors: the cultural subordination of patients; their limited competence and resources; and their organisational weakness. All have now changed. The cultural subordination of patients was linked to the ascendancy of scientific medicine. The decades immediately after the Second World War were the golden age of scientific authority in health care. The medical profession enjoyed immense cultural authority, an authority partly derived from its association with science. That authority was strengthened by the great advances in the application of high technology solutions to illness, advances stimulated, as we have seen, by the demands of war: consider the discussion above of the transformation of the pharmaceutical industry and the emergence of sophisticated technologies of diagnostic imaging. Starr's words about the United States could be more widely generalised. He writes that the connection with science gave the medical profession 'an especially persuasive claim to authority. Unlike the law and clergy, it enjoys close bonds with modern science, and at least for most of the last century, scientific knowledge has held a privileged status in the hierarchy of belief' (Starr, 1982: 4).

That cultural authority on the side of doctors was mirrored by incompetence among most patients. It was not simply that patients deferred to doctors; even in circumstances where they might have wished to challenge medical authority they did not have the necessary skills or information to do so. The flow of clinical information, the nature of medical record keeping, the esoteric discourse about medical issues in a specialised scientific language: all worked against assertiveness on the part of patients.

Finally, the organisation of health care systems was biased against patients and in favour of professional elites. On one side the medical profession had a reservoir of institutional capital, embodied in the rich and well-organised professional associations that across most industrial nations represented doctors' interests. In many nations professional interests had organised and struck bargains about the allocation of regulatory authority with states before the emergence of democratic politics (for a case study, see Brazier *et al.*, 1993). The authority of doctors rested on institutional residues from a predemocratic age. Patients, by contrast, had little: no inheritance of institutions, no obvious source of organisational leadership, no helpful technologies of organisational mobilisation. Even in systems where there had once been a tradition of patient organisation – such as in the German-based sickness funds – those organisations had, by the postwar years, become professionalised oligarchies.

If we take the above as a summary of conditions in the decade after the end of Second World War, then a summary of conditions in the 1990s will help us get some sense of the changes that have come about. The institutional world of patient politics has changed. Although there are no systematic databases available which would allow us to demonstrate the observation, all the scattered evidence across a range of jurisdictions points strongly in one direction: patients are no longer a poorly organised group. The rise of patient organisation has taken two particularly important forms. The first is the spread of patient self-help groups, notably those uniting patients linked by common chronic complaints. The second is the development of health advocacy coalitions. I believe the trends identified by Peterson for the United States are part of a wider international movement. He writes:

> At the risk of oversimplifying a complex evolutionary process, one can describe the health care representational community as having travelled through three distinct stages of development. Until the 1940s and probably through the 1950s era of reform debate it conformed with the definition of a block community. The 1960s and 1970s saw it become more dyadic, as new stake-challenger groups increasingly polarized health care politics while stakeholders maintained their old alliance. The stresses produced by the 1980s and early 1990s have made stakeholders more competitive with one another, while time and opportunity have increased the number and resilience of stake-challengers, creating a heterogeneous representational network.
>
> (Peterson, 1993: 413)

These changes are general across the advanced industrial world because they reflect developments which are not unique to health care systems or to the United States; they are part of wider changes in the character of group mobilisation in democratic polities. Some are due to the altered technology of mobilisation: the development of both 'soft' technologies (new techniques of mass communication, such as mail shots) and of 'hard' technologies (based on electronics) which make it easier for policy 'entrepreneurs' to bring groups into existence. Some are due to an increase in the propensity to mobilise, connected to rising levels of education, and therefore competence, among populations.

Some are due to the decline of a major competitor in the market for activists, political parties, whose mass active support has shown a long term fall.

The factors that have affected the capacity of patients to mobilise are also changing their resources and competence. Some of the influences at work include the rising levels of formal education encountered by doctors when treating patients, and the spread of information about illness and treatments (for instance through a lay press that now, much more than a generation ago, reports medical matters). An unremarked element in this transformation is the changed character of encounters between male doctors and women. The importance of these encounters lies not only in the role of women as patients, but also in their roles as carers: as mothers of the young, daughters of the old, and siblings of the sick, women's caring roles provide an added set of opportunities for encounters with doctors. It is undeniable that doctors encountering women in the 1990s are encountering more self-confident, better educated and less deferential cohorts than faced the doctors of the 1940s.

The decline in the cultural authority of medicine is also connected to wider social changes. The evidence about the declining authority of the physician is widespread. It includes: the spread of 'self-help' therapies; the growing tendency of patients to sue doctors; the sort of revolts against doctor-controlled rationing which Saltman and von Otter (1992) traced as a main point of pressure in the rise of the managed market in the command and control Scandinavian systems. These changes in turn reflect wider alterations in democratic politics: the rise of consumer-led pressure groups; changes in the felt competence of citizens when faced with professionals; and the spread of information about treatment options through a free media increasingly devoting space to medical matters.

The systems of universalism created in the decades after the Second World War worked by overriding the market: the whole point of the entitlement system was that it allocated health care as a mark of citizenship. That could not mean, of course, that there was no system of allocation: the offer of health care as a free or nearly free service at the point of consumption meant that some means of rationing had to be devised. The history of health care systems, almost from the moment of the creation of entitlements, was a history of struggle with this problem: the creation of residual market mechanisms, such as charges for some pharmaceuticals, was a sign of that struggle. The character of democratic politics, however, was a considerable help in resource allocation. Formally pluralist political systems were actually characterised by inequalities in the ability of different interests to mobilise in the political arena, and by the persistence of hierarchies and cultural patterns dating from predemocratic eras. Doctors, an interest group forged for the most part before the emergence of formally democratic politics, were major beneficiaries of this state of affairs, notably in their dealings with patients. They enjoyed organisational advantages, cultural hegemony and control over resources like information. This meant that doctors could occupy a central role in gatekeeping, in regulating the demands of patients for health care.

It is a truism of health care politics that this system of control has been significantly weakened by the changes summarised above: the declining cultural authority of doctors, the rising sense of competence among patients, and the changing institutional landscapes of health care systems. These changes are not unique to health care: they reflect wider changes which have come over capitalist democracies. In some instances there is an intersection between political organisation and economic mechanisms. The great success of capitalist economies in the decades after the Second World War greatly increased the disposable income of citizens. In particular it expanded large and prosperous middle classes. Many of the rigidities identified by observers of 'command' health care systems, like Saltman, are the result of demands by these newly prosperous groups. Health care is famously a merit good, the demand for which rises with income. The stresses and strains in the command systems came from prosperous groups enriched by the 'long boom' demanding the right to 'top up' citizenship entitlements by buying supplementary services: better hospital facilities, speedier elective surgery than the public system could deliver, treatment such as psychiatric services often not available as public entitlements. Market ideologies served the strategic interests of a wide range of different groups: sections of the middle class demanding the right to use their economic resources to buy additions to citizenship entitlements; state actors anxious to use market disciplines to control patient demand as more traditional systems of control were eroded; entrepreneurs ready to satisfy demands not met by publicly funded providers.

Markets, empowerment and subordination

Any social order worth its salt will be riddled with tensions and contradictions, because a social order of any worth will simultaneously try to empower and to control numerous different interests. The history of health care is a history of contradiction and tension. The entitlement systems developed across the advanced capitalist world after the Second World War were expressions of the ideology of democratic citizenship, but their operation relied on control mechanisms which were predemocratic in origin. The dynamism of capitalism and the spread of democratic organisation in turn undermined those controls. The rise of market ideology has occurred because it can be appropriated by a range of different interests. In this lies both its strength and its weakness: it promises different things to different people, but not all the promises can be reconciled. Three sources of tension are worth stressing.

First, market ideology simultaneously holds out prospects of empowerment and of subordination. For many groups of patients – notably those with the capacity to buy access to medical care, either directly or through their employers – it offers power: the power to appropriate resources and the power to challenge hitherto dominant medical professionals as the 'patient-customer'. For some providers it also offers the prospect of empowerment: consider the use made by GPs in Britain of the fundholding system to change the balance between themselves and consultants. For institutional purchasers of care, on the other hand, market ideologies legitimise mechanisms of control: over patients, by cost sharing; over professional deliverers of care, by competition that squeezes more effort and compliance out of the health care workforce.

A second source of tension takes us back to the different environments in which health care systems are embedded: the economic and the political, the capitalist and the democratic. It has been said of the American health care system that it attempts to 'embed a Schumpeterian health economy within a populist political culture' (Robinson, 1996: 156). We might say more generally that health care systems in the advanced industrial nations attempt to mix Schumpeter's economy with democratic politics: on the one side a world of corporate power, of eternal creative destruction through competitive innovation, of large institutional hierarchies managed alongside nation states; on the other side, the egalitarian institutions of democratic citizenship. Two worlds, of institutional control and individual empowerment, live uneasily together.

That tension is connected to a third, which is geopolitical. It will be obvious that the political (democratic) settings into which health care institutions are embedded are mostly national in scope. The strategic calculations by key actors – interest groups mobilising to influence policy, politicians manoeuvring to win elections – have to be made within the confines of nationally organised political institutions. The economic setting, equally as obvious, is international, even on occasions global in reach: the strategic calculations of key actors, like firms, have to be made in the realisation that success has to be achieved in arenas that transcend national boundaries. Many actors straddle the worlds of the national and the global. For some particularly important actors – democratically elected governments – straddling those worlds is the essence of their job.

References

Alber, J. (1988) 'Is there a crisis of the welfare state? Cross-national evidence from Europe, North America and Japan', *European Sociological Review*, **4** (3): 181–207.

Alford, R. (1975) *Health Care Politics: Ideological and Interest Group Barriers to Reform*, Chicago: University of Chicago Press.

Banta, H.D. (1980) 'The diffusion of the computed tomography (CT) scanner in the United States', *International Journal of Health Services*, **10** (2): 251–69.

Brazier, M, Lovecy, J, Moran, M, and Potton, M. (1993) 'Falling from a tightrope: Doctors and lawyers between the market and the state', *Political Studies*, **41** (2): 215–32.

Chollet, D. (1994) 'Employer-based health insurance in a changing work force', *Health Affairs*, **13** (1): 315–26.

Ferrera, M. (1995) 'The rise and fall of democratic universalism: Health care reform in Italy, 1978–94', *Journal of Health Politics, Policy and Law*, **20** (2): 275–302.

Foote, S. (1992) *Managing the Medical Arms Race: Public Policy and Medical Device Innovation*, Berkeley: University of California Press.

Jencks, S. and Schieber, G. (1991) 'Containing US health costs: What bullet to bite?', *Health Care Financing Review*, Annual Supplement, 1–12.

Lotz, P. (1993) 'Demand as a driving force in medical innovation', *International Journal of Technology Assessment in Health Care*, **9** (2): 174–88.

Maynard. A. (1995) 'Health care reform: Don't confuse me with the facts, stupid!' in *Conference Report: Four Country Conference on Health Care Reforms and Health Policies in the United States, Canada, Germany and the Netherlands*, 23–5 February 1995, Amsterdam-Rotterdam, The Hague: Ministry of Health, Welfare and Sport, pp. 47–57.

Moran, M. (1995) 'Explaining change in the National Health Service: Corporatism, closure and democratic capitalism', *Public Policy and Administration*, **10** (2): 21–33.

Morone, J. (1990) *The Democratic Wish*, New York: Basic Books.

Organisation for Economic Cooperation and Development (1987) *Financing and Delivering Health Care*, Paris: OECD.

Organisation for Economic Cooperation and Development (1992) *The Reform of Health Care: A Comparative Analysis of Seven OECD Countries*, Paris: OECD.

Peterson, M. (1993) 'Political influence in the 1990s: From iron triangles to policy networks', *Journal of Health Politics, Policy and Law*, **18** (2): 395–438.

Reinhardt, U. (1989) 'Health care spending and American competitiveness', *Health Affairs*, **8** (4): 5–21.

Robinson, J. (1996) 'The dynamics and limits of corporate growth in health care', *Health Affairs*, **15** (2): 155–69.

Saltman, R. and von Otter, C. (1992) *Planned Markets and Public Competition*, Buckingham: Open University Press.

Sharp, A. (ed.) (1994) *Leap Into the Dark: The Changing Role of the State in New Zealand since 1984*, Auckland: Auckland University Press.

Starr, P. (1982) *The Social Transformation of American Medicine*, New York: Basic Books.

Temin, H. (1980) *Taking your Medicine*, Cambridge, Massachusetts: Harvard University Press.

Trajtenberg, M. (1990) *Economic Analysis of Product Innovation: The Case of CT Scanners*, Cambridge, Massachusetts: Harvard University Press.

World Bank (1993) *Investing in Health. World Development Report 1993*, Washington, DC: The World Bank.

I gave an earlier version of this chapter to the workshop at the University of Northumbria, June 1996, where the drafts of chapters for this volume were outlined and discussed. It is a pleasure to acknowledge the many helpful comments and criticisms from my collaborators. I should mention in particular Wendy Ranade for her editorial guidance, Ted

Marmor who gave me the volume containing the Maynard reference, and Michael Hill who, though not a contributor to the volume, was an invaluable participant in the workshop.

CHAPTER 3

Economic perspectives on markets and health care

JOHN APPLEBY

Introduction

For more than a generation most of the health care industry in the UK
has been run along the lines of a command and control economy. In the
rather negative language of economics, the NHS has represented a gross
distortion in the health care market, introducing monopolies in production and monopsonies in labour markets (backed by government legislation), and substituting a form of central planning in place of market-
determined prices for the allocation of health care services. Monopolies,
monopsonies, the absence of prices and the confused distinction between 'consumers' and 'producers' are the stuff of nightmares for free
marketeers. But such 'distortions' were *deliberate* (and popular) responses to a health care 'system' that was widely perceived to have failed to
deliver what people wanted.

Over 40 years after the introduction of the NHS (and with perhaps
only dim memories of the reasons for its creation) there was a perception – more particularly a government perception – that the NHS was
failing on a number of fronts. It was seen to be bureaucratic and unresponsive to the needs of patients; the producers of health care were felt
to have usurped the sovereignty of 'consumers'; and in particular, it was
thought to lack the right incentive structures to pursue the efficient production of health care. The origins of the 1991 reforms of the NHS can
also be traced back to the political spirit and philosophy of Conservative administrations throughout the 1980s (Butler, 1994). While the
1991 NHS reforms introduced a number of changes, perhaps the most
audacious and revolutionary was the creation of an internal or quasi-
market, the origins of which are most commonly attributed to Alain Enthoven (see, for example, Enthoven, 1985). Detaching the providers of
health care from their guaranteed budgets and leaving them to compete
for business from (the still state-attached) purchasers was seen to be the
way to introduce new incentives to promote efficiency and choice in the
NHS.

This (short) tale of health care policy in the UK is not unique (as
other chapters in this book testify). Indeed, at the risk of overgeneralisa-
tion, the idea of some form of quasi, regulated or managed health care
market in the public sector is probably now as globally pervasive as the
policy of privatisation and the divestment of public assets in general.

How market ideology and specifically, market tools, have been applied in different countries has depended on existing structures and organisations and on country-specific perceptions of the problems that such change is hoped to resolve. Despite variations in implementation detail, the new economic environments being created in health care around the world are often grounded in economic theory and the conclusions economists (some defunct) have drawn from their examination of economic relationships.

Such examination has suggested that markets can be useful mechanisms for getting to grips with the complex business of producing and allocating goods and services. Moreover, they are seen – and not just by economists – as often providing the right economic environment to promote productive efficiency on the supply side and maximisation (subject to purchasing power) of consumers' utility on the demand side. Markets can also be viewed as instruments which, by a combination of evolution and deliberate design, provide a forum for rationing resources (and hence goods and services) which, due to the demands placed upon them, are nearly always in short supply.

But the choice facing health care policy makers is not simply between command or market economy. Rather (and as our experience suggests), it is about a balance between control and freedom, with the aim of moving towards the objectives we specify for our health care systems. Different countries face this choice from different starting points, cultural perspectives and institutional organisations. Moreover, the answers to some basic social value questions, as noted by Fuchs (1974: 12) – 'What kind of people are we? What kind of life do we want to lead? What kind of society do we want to build for our children and grandchildren? How much weight do we want to put on individual freedom? How much to equality? … ' – are essential in shaping our health care system. Different countries will have different answers, making the pursuit of some health care policies more acceptable than others.

This chapter attempts a critical description of the economic rationale underpinning the choices which many countries are now taking with respect to their health care systems: namely, the use of market tools and/or the creation or strengthening of regulatory systems for managing markets. The overarching theme is not the dichotomous and mutually exclusive division between market and nonmarket economic environments, or a view of change based on a continuous path. Rather, the theme is one of action and reaction, of pendulum swings in policy and attempts to forge a composite health care economy employing market and nonmarket tools and processes.

The chapter begins with a restatement of what economists mean by the term market and in particular their view of market efficiency in general. It then looks at the characteristics of health care as an economic commodity and the extent to which it 'fits' into the traditional economic framework of a market and the theoretical predictions of market failure. Next, the chapter describes various forms of market structure and regulation implemented in response to perceived failures in both market and nonmarket systems. The final sections deal with subsequent issues arising from the use of markets (and more accurately, market tools) in health care, in particular, the nature of competition on the supply and demand sides and overall market regulation.

Efficient markets

For most commodities and under certain conditions, markets can provide an efficient or optimal solution to the problem of allocating scarce resources. This statement is qualified: *most* (not all) commodities; *certain* (not all) conditions; *can* (not will) provide an efficient solution. It also raises the question of what we consider to be *optimal* or *efficient*. Before looking at the archetypal economic conditions for markets to reach an equilibrium (in which allocations are deemed to be efficient) it is important to be clear what is meant by an efficient allocation.

For economists, optimality or efficiency in this context is usually defined in terms articulated by the Italian social scientist Vilfredo Pareto (1971). In Paretian terms, an efficient allocation of resources is achieved when no single individual can be made better off without making someone else worse off. Along with Pareto's other views – that individuals are the best judges of their own welfare, and that a society's total welfare is merely the sum of each individual's utility – the optimality criterion should be seen as a value judgement, and not necessarily as how things are or how they should be (see, for example, Mishan, 1981). Pareto's value judgements are attempts to provide reference points or a 'framework on the world around us to give it order and meaning' (Cullis and Jones, 1992: 2–3). Other views – sociological, psychological, and so on – are of course just as valid; here, however, Pareto's judgements are taken as the economic starting point in describing the almost universal human experience of markets.

In the frictionless and knowledgeable environment of the perfect market, the demands of consumers and the activities of producers are brought together – indeed, reconciled – through prices. Within the assumed objective of the maximisation of their utility, consumers make judgements about their level of demand based on the value they expect to derive from commodities and their ability and willingness to pay. Demand is thus a function not only of consumers' desires (or perceived needs or wants) *but also of their wealth*. Producers – within the assumed objective of maximisation of profits – adjust their production within the prevailing price for their product so that the production costs of the last unit produced is equal to the market price for that commodity.

The outcome of production and consumption decisions is a market-clearing price, a particular aggregate level of production (which matches aggregate levels of consumption), a particular level of profit and a particular level of utility enjoyed by consumers. Moreover, the outcome is deemed to be efficient: producers produce at minimum cost (given competition), all inputs are used as efficiently as possible, and it is impossible to increase output (making one person better off) without reducing it elsewhere. And, given the market clearing price, typical consumers cannot make themselves better off (by choosing to buy more than the equilibrium price implies they should) without somehow inducing producers to make themselves worse off.

This simple view of market exchange leading to an efficient allocation of goods and services depends on a raft of assumptions. These include: the single-minded maximisation of utility and profit on the part of consumers and producers respectively; the ability of consumers to judge best their own welfare and the benefits they could derive from commodities; the ability of producers to adjust production in the light of a correct understanding of market conditions; the independence of supply and demand; the inability of individual consumers or producers to significantly affect prices; and the absence of externalities (the imposition on some third party, without their choice, of a benefit or cost as a result of a decision by some other consumer or producer in a market).

Failed markets

The conditions/assumptions needed for a market to reach a Paretian efficient equilibrium are extensive and significant. In fact there are an infinite number of examples where these conditions are *not* met, to the extent that markets either fail to develop at all, only develop in a very limited way, or fail to produce an efficient allocation. There is an analogy with the evolutionary process for living things. Under certain environmental conditions some organisms find it impossible to survive while others mutate and develop to find an environmental niche. What is then observed (by definition) are the successes; complete failures are never observed (again by definition); and partial successes are only observed fleetingly as they mature then decline into oblivion as environmental conditions prevail. Because failures are never (or only rarely) observed, the impression can be gained that the process (evolution) is inherently and uniquely good at producing living things. In fact, it is also a process that produces numerous failures.

The point to draw from this analogy is not that markets are in some way akin to the 'natural order' of things, universally applicable and in some way representing a fundamental baseline in economic and human activity, but that markets are much more likely to *fail* to deliver an efficient solution to the problem of the allocation of scarce resources than they are to *succeed*. Moreover, protecting certain market failures may be desirable, just as protecting certain animals is seen as desirable despite their failure to cope with prevailing environmental conditions.

Health care is just one example which is widely seen as an economic commodity which cannot, or should not, be traded within traditional market structures. There are two issues here, contingent on 'can' and 'should'. These relate respectively to the *feasibility* of trading health care efficiently in a market and the *desirability* of doing so. Both are interrelated, but are worth treating separately.

The problems with the ability of a traditional market mechanism to produce an efficient allocation in health care stem primarily (though not exclusively) from information asymmetries or 'informational impactedness' (cf. Williamson, 1973). Apart from the fact that when ill, potential consumers of health care are unlikely to be able to choose rationally, the lack of information and knowledge on the part of the consumer is such that the very notion of consumer sovereignty is undermined. This is not always and everywhere the case; health care is not a homogenous product. By and large, health care consumption decisions concerning a headache or toothache are much easier to take and accommodate within the framework of expected utility theory than for a broken leg. However, it is also true to say that in many ways health care is an extremely customised product, dependent not only on the type of illness, but the type of person with the illness and the type of person delivering the care.

Nevertheless, informational problems on the consumer side suggest that rational decision making is undermined to the extent that the traditional axioms underpinning consumer sovereignty – completeness, transitivity and selection – are all contravened. If consumers find it difficult, if not impossible, to rank their preferences for health care (and other) goods and services (completeness); or, because of this, cannot produce logical orderings of consumption preferences of the form: if A is preferred to B, and B to C, then A is preferred to C (transitivity); or, partly as a consequence, are unable to decide on their preferred state of health, then there are clearly problems at the heart of the market mechanism. A common solution to this source of market failure has and largely remains the creation of a knowledgeable agent able to act on the consumers' behalf, the doctor. However, this solution produces further problems. In particular the potential linking of supply and demand through the opportunity the agency relationship provides for the exploitation of consumers by producers, or 'supplier-induced demand' (Evans, 1974). In turn, this problem is implicitly recognised through the creation of an ethical framework governing the practice of medicine.

Additional problems stemming from the nature of health and health care abound. Williamson (1973) identified a number of conditions which, if dominant in any transaction process (which may occur in a market setting, but not necessarily), suggest that transaction costs can escalate to the point where markets start to fail. Some of Williamson's conditions have already been alluded to (e.g. informational impactedness, potential supplier opportunism and the limits to consumer knowledge). In addition, there are problems associated with the complexity of the consumer's decision process, the considerable uncertainty surrounding the timing of ill health, the (usually) small number of individual transactions involved in health care for individual consumers which makes it hard to arrive at an agreed market clearing price, and the complications of the source of utility consumers derive from a health care transaction. This latter problem refers to the existence of utility derived from the *process* of consuming health care and not just utility derived as a *consequence* of health care consumption.

An important complication in the operation of conventional markets is the almost ubiquitous existence of uncertainty in health care. The unpredictability of illness and hence future consumption of health care, plus uncertainties about the type and cost of health care, make it a prime candidate for an insurance market. But while insurance markets can, through the spreading of risk, help to reduce welfare losses (by easing access to health care at the time of need by effectively reducing prices) failures can arise.

Moral hazard may occur when individuals (faced with much reduced prices at the time of consumption) may overconsume health care relative to their needs. To an extent this problem can be ameliorated by the professional conduct of clinicians plus an effective increase in prices consumers face through the use of deductibles and co-insurance. However, moral hazard can also imply a failure on the part of consumers to seek out the best deal in the market, as one of the key incentives – prices – is not functioning properly. Therefore, the competitive mechanism for suppliers fails to function efficiently as consumers have little incentive to shop around.

Adverse selection can also arise as a consequence of information asymmetries in health care insurance markets. The efficiency of insurance agents to discriminate effectively on the basis of actuarial risk is hampered by the fact that consumers tend to know more about their health state than do insurers. High risk groups should in theory face higher premiums than low risk groups. But if there is adverse selection then the pooling of risks is affected, resulting in the wrong premium levels being set. In attempting to overcome this problem, insurance agents try to identify high risk groups (using, for example, factors related to ill health, or potential ill health, such as age). The failure of (private) medical insurance markets to provide adequate coverage is evident in all countries where such markets exist. The most notable gaps in coverage tend to occur for high risk groups such as the elderly and the poor.

Monopoly is a potential problem in all markets, but for insurance markets there is a strong tendency towards monopoly due to the increasing returns to scale arising from maximising the risk pool. Although larger risk pools enable insurers to cover claims in relation to premiums, monopoly also provides an incentive to exploit consumers.

As in conventional health care markets, these insurance market failures have led to the implementation of nonmarket solutions such as the creation of governmental institutions or interventions to improve access to health care. In the United States the intervention has taken the form of state-run insurance schemes such as Medicare and Medicaid. In other countries social insurance – although perhaps run independently of government – are regulated to ensure that, for example, adverse selection is minimised.

It is worth noting at this point that health care is not being classed as a unique commodity; there are many others which also fail to fit into the constraints of expected utility theory and lead to allocatively inefficient solutions within a market context. The point to note, however, is that health care, as McGuire *et al.* (1992) state, is towards the untypical end of a spectrum of goods and services which fail, to varying degrees, to fit.

Finally, market failure can be seen in a wider way to encompass a potential failing with regard to a widely held concern in health care, namely equity. The consumption and production outcomes of markets rely on the willingness and ability of consumers to pay. Crucially, the ability to express demand through the ability to pay is curtailed when (as is often the case in health care) incomes are too low to cover prices. In this case the market will attribute a lower valuation to care needed by the poor than to care demanded by the rich. This situation is not unique to health care, and would generally not be seen as an example of market failure. However, even if all the intricate preconditions for an efficient market allocation hold in health care, the resulting market-derived distribution is simply undesirable for many people, as it will be partly based on the ability to pay, and in almost all societies wealth is unevenly distributed (in most, grossly so). In effect, the market has not been given the right signals in order to produce a distribution of health care that most people desire for themselves and, importantly, for others. This outcome can be corrected – through, for example, redistributing income – but the fact remains that the market *inherently* cannot cope with the almost universal human concern for the welfare of others.

For some, 'multi-tiered' (i.e. inequitable) systems are seen as a positive boon to the poor compared with single-tiered systems. For example, Enthoven (1994) adopts a trickle-down view of health care in which those parts of the system used by the rich will produce innovations in quality and service which are eventually taken up by parts of the system serving the poor. This argument has also been used to justify differences in the speed of access to secondary care of GP fundholders' patients compared with nonfundholders' in the UK. Clearly, this is an empirical argument as well as an ethical one, and one which merely serves to point out that there *may* be trade-offs involved between equity and quality. As Fuchs (1974) would note, the ethical component of this issue concerns the values we attach to such (often conflicting) concepts as personal freedom, choice, community solidarity, and so on. The answers to these social value questions vary from country to country and over time.

The use of markets and market tools in health care

Given the unusual degree of consensus among economists that health care is generally an unsuitable commodity to be traded in a market, the apparent popularity among policy makers for market-based solutions to perceived problems in health care may seem surprising. However, as the case studies described in subsequent chapters illustrate, policy makers have played a subtler and more sophisticated game than the crude, wholesale imposition of competitive market structures on health care systems.

In general, the reasons for this policy selectivity stem from the desire to avoid or ameliorate market failures in health care (whilst trying to address perceived public sector failures) and the fact that market *tools* can be applied to *parts* of health care systems and do not have to be all-encompassing. Together with a perception that certain parts of a system work and deliver an acceptable outcome, while others do not, there has tended to be a desire for partial rather than total reform. Perhaps to many policy makers' relief, Alain Enthoven provided a possible prescription – the internal market – which potentially offered a model of a pluralistic health care system combining market and nonmarket features. In addition, there are practical realities which cannot be ignored; policy makers do not start with a clean slate, for example. There are many combinations and permutations for organising and funding health care systems and all health care systems are (to a greater or lesser extent) pluralistic in terms of their organisation, ownership and financing (Maxwell, 1988). Where systems can move is constrained – at least in the short to medium term – by where they start from. Furthermore, there are a whole variety of policy implementation barriers arising from historic patterns of professional power, and political and public acceptability regarding change.

In practice, therefore, the recourse to market-based solutions to perceived problems in health care systems has been piecemeal rather than total. And in general, the opportunities for markets have been limited. The opportunities that do exist arise from two areas in health care systems: supply and intermediate demand. Figure 3.1 (based on OECD, 1992) illustrates a typical health care system made up of three groups: consumers/the general population, primary and secondary health care providers and the intermediaries (health care agents). Intermediaries may be private or voluntary/charitable insurance organisations or the state (through powers invested in its representatives). Funding in the system may be initially raised in a variety of ways (through general or specific taxes, for example) and channelled to providers also in a variety of ways (fee for item of service, preset global budgets etc.) in exchange for health care services. Consumers may also pay directly out of pocket for health care. All health care systems utilise a combination of funding methods (perhaps tending towards one method rather than another) and all tend to have a mix of public, private and voluntary

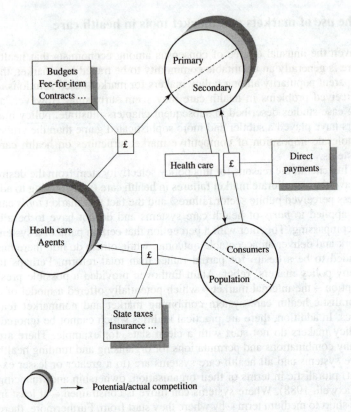

Figure 3.1 **Archetypal health care system**

suppliers and agents, again, tending towards one or two particular types.

At one competitive extreme (and in the absence of insurance markets), Figure 3.1 reduces to Figure 3.2. However, no recent market-based health care reform has gone this far. Rather, the choice of where to introduce competitive markets and their scope and organisation has been guided by perceptions/evidence of particular problems (cost containment, poor access, macroeconomic demands for greater efficiency etc.) and a recognition that wholesale reform of all aspects of health care systems is simply uncalled for. In addition, as noted earlier, the extent of reform introduced is also constrained by the degree of political, professional and public propensity to accept change. Moreover, the process of change itself can be costly depending on initial organisational structures. The costs of moving from one type of system to another are likely to influence at least short-term changes (see, for example, Ludbrook and Maynard, 1988, concerning their critique of social insurance).

Although the potential configuration of market-based environments is vast, particularly in the domain of the intermediate demand or health

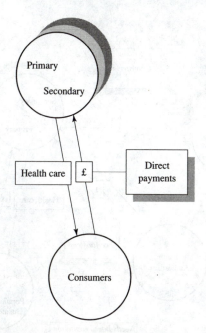

Figure 3.2   **Competitive health care market with no insurance**

agent – as illustrated by Figures 3.3 and 3.4, showing the essence of the newly reformed systems in the UK and the Netherlands – all countries which have undertaken market-based reforms have either introduced or in some way strengthened competition in the supply of health care.

For countries with particularly dominant health care agents, a traditional lack of experience among consumers of dealing directly with health care providers, or in which there is a general ethos of passive rather than active consumers – such as in the UK – there has tended to be a more limited use of market tools in this sector of the system. Wherever competition has been introduced, there are a number of problems which can arise on the supply and/or demand side of the market, and in the overall market management and regulation of new arrangements. Some of these issues are explored below.

Supply side issues

The introduction or enhancement of competition on the supply side has been a common policy among countries which have implemented market-based reforms of their health care systems. However, the move to competition among suppliers is not straightforward and raises a number

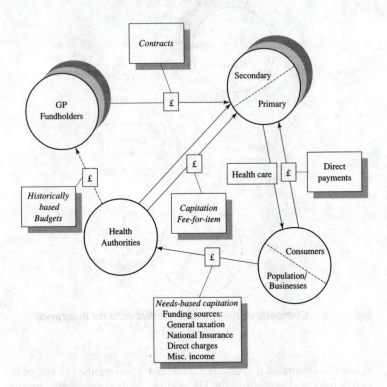

Figure 3.3 **UK, post-reform, public health care system**

of economic issues related to the degree of competition created and the impact on nonefficiency objectives of health care systems such as access and quality.

An important criticism of internal markets – particularly where they have been introduced in countries where one of the traditional objects of policy has been to create localised monopolies for reasons of cost effectiveness – is the lack of competition. In a health care world in which decades of planning has tried to ensure that duplication of provision is minimised, what scope is there for purchaser choice and provider competition?

To take one step back, and using the UK as an example, it appears that it is actually quite difficult to establish a robust and accurate measure of the degree of competition in the system. Traditional industrial concentration measures (such as the Hirschman–Herfindahl Index, Miller, 1982) which have been calculated (Appleby *et al.*, 1991) for a single specialty (general surgery) across one Regional Health Authority in the UK suggest that a significant number of hospitals do in fact face a

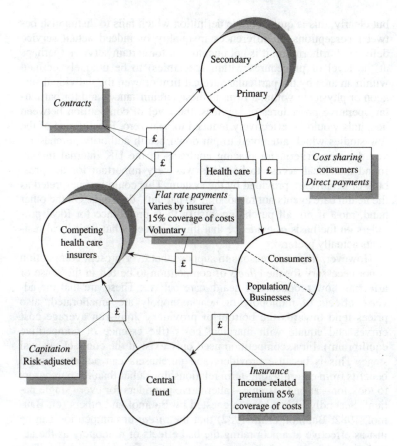

Figure 3.4 **Dutch, post-reform, health care system**

level of competition, and would be regarded as nonmonopolies under antitrust rules applied by the US Department of Justice. It has also been estimated that in the major conurbations of the UK, only 8 per cent of all acute providers have *no* competitors within a thirty minute travel distance for specialties such as general surgery, orthopaedics, ENT and gynaecology (Propper, 1995). Similar work for New Zealand has revealed similar results (Ashton and Press, 1997).

However, these estimates need to be interpreted with great care. Although there is evidence to suggest that patients, hypothetically, would be willing to trade off travel time for quicker treatment (hence potentially increasing the number of health care providers in competition for patients), it is not clear how willing this trade-off becomes in practice. Moreover, there are problems with defining the 'product' that patients are either willing to travel for, or that hospitals are providing. Both the studies noted above used the specialty as the unit of health care product;

but clearly, this is quite a crude definition which fails to distinguish between perceptions of differences in quality or indeed actual service
delivery. Furthermore, it is not uncommon for certain services (perhaps
at the level of procedures within specialties) to be uniquely defined
within an area by the particular surgical firm or even the individual sur-
geon or physician within a firm. In these circumstances and for particular operative procedures or services, the level of competition between
hospitals would be effectively reduced to near zero. Finally, one of the
few studies which attempted to pin down health authority purchasers'
key decision criteria for placing contracts in the UK internal market
found that local access to hospitals was very important for the great
bulk of health care provided by the system. This could be interpreted as
the health care agents not responding to patients' demands. On the other
hand, most if not all purchasers justify their preference for local providers on the basis of evidence that this is indeed what their local residents actually prefer.

However, there are reasons to suppose that ever-present competition
is not necessary for the *effects* of competition to be felt in the sense of
affecting how producers of health care behave. These are that the adverse effects of monopoly or near-monopoly are ameliorated; also
prices tend towards the bottom of providers' long-run average cost
curves and equate with marginal costs (the essence of competitive
equilibrium). First, competition need only exist at the contract renewal
stage. This is because providers and purchasers can achieve mutual
benefits from entering long-term relationships rather than for purchasers
to look for – at one extreme – alternative providers for every single patient. Secondly, it has been suggested by Baumol and others (cf. Baumol, 1982; Baumol, *et al.* 1982) that the *threat* of competition can be
just as effective at ameliorating the bad effects of monopoly as the actual or literal physical presence of competing firms in a market. This
notion of contestability rests primarily on the cost side of the market
and crucially requires that there is freedom of entry to and exit from the
market. Moreover, it also relies on a certain behavioural pattern of
(technical) monopolists under threat of possible competition from new
entrants to a market. Given the sunk costs necessary in the set up of a
new hospital, any lags in the time it takes for new competitors to enter a
market could persuade current hospitals to extract monopoly rent while
the going is easy, the opposite effect proposed by contestability theory.
Clearly, a static analysis of contestability is insufficient to predict the
reactions of providers in a dynamic market. Over time, purchasers are
vulnerable to 'provider capture' so, initially low-cost new entrants may
tend to exert monopoly pressure on their purchasers in the same way as
the original providers.

Although the conditions for contestability may not be always and
everywhere in place, there is evidence that purchasers in the UK internal market are testing the potential level of competition through increasing use of tendering for clinical services. To date tendering has been at

the margins in terms of the value of contracts let this way (Appleby, 1995) but it is one way for purchasers simultaneously to signal to current providers their willingness to switch to alternative suppliers and also to indicate to potential new entrants the likely business opportunities of entering a new market. Given the time scales involved in entering and exiting the health care market, it is likely to take some years before we are clear of the actual effects of contestability, including the actual behaviour and reactions of existing providers in technically monopolistic markets.

Demand side issues

Two particular, though related, economic issues arise on the demand/health agent sector of health care systems in relation to market-based reforms. First, there is the interaction between the demanders (whether consumers or health agents) and suppliers in systems with competitive provision of health care. Secondly, there are issues arising in systems which introduce competition between health agents.

The theoretical benefits arising from competition in the supply of health care are highly dependent on the behaviour of actors on the demand side of the market. The key motivating factor for suppliers to improve their performance is the potential threat of losing business if they fail to respond appropriately to the demands/needs of either consumers, or agents acting on their behalf. However, this motivating force depends in turn on the incentives faced by consumers or health agents encouraging them actively to seek out good performance and to employ the ultimate consumer sanction of moving their business elsewhere.

In a system in which there are no health care agents – simply end-users or consumers dealing directly with suppliers – then the incentive reduces to a desire to obtain the best outcome for the out-of-pocket expense. But, as noted earlier, the health care consumer is faced with a raft of problems when confronted with the need to make the right purchasing choice. These include: the lack of information as to the outcome of care delivered by alternative suppliers, uncertainty as to when care will be needed, and difficulties in assessing the outcome of care after the event. All these problems make the consumer in this situation a rather weak actor in exerting the right pressure on suppliers to improve performance and hence reap the benefits markets can in theory provide.

Some of these problems can be partly solved in systems which employ agents whose job it is to represent consumers. However, the use of agents does not necessarily guarantee that suppliers will be faced with the appropriate incentives to minimise their costs, maximise productive efficiency, and so on. Agents – whether government organisations or private/independent insurance firms – can, for example, face many of the information asymmetries confronting individual consumers. Moreover, it is not clear whether such agents necessarily face the *right* incentives to perform their purchasing role efficiently, exploiting opportunities created by competition between suppliers. This may be especially true when consumers only exert negligible influence over their agents through some competitive mechanism (such as being able to select agents). Where competitive pressures on health agents are absent – as in the UK with district health authorities – agents invariably face an alternative set of traditional public sector performance incentives set by government. Whether these are any worse, better or the same as competition in motivating agents to exert pressure on suppliers is unclear and will largely depend on the sort of incentives employed and the rigor with which they are enforced (Appleby, 1996).

The potential 'incentive deficit' facing health care agents tied into a traditional government bureaucracy is susceptible to influence by markets, however. For example, a greater degree of sovereignty can be extended to consumers of health care by introducing choice as to their representative agent (such as in the Netherlands). To be effective, this choice needs to carry with it the ability to transfer funds from one agent to another and for agents to be in such a position that the shifting of funds out of their control is considered an important loss. In effect, these are the sorts of incentives facing private medical insurance firms. However, without robust regulation, the requirement for compulsory coverage, cover for those unable to pay for insurance and an ability of insurers to select good suppliers over bad, such a system fails to deliver on a whole range of health care objectives from efficiency and equity, to cost-effective care and adequate coverage. This has been the experience in the USA for decades. Moreover, depending on how the system is designed, there can be substantial transaction costs involved in operating such a system of direct consumer choice.

In the UK the introduction of budgets held by GPs (GP fundholders), coupled with the traditional freedom to choose a GP, has provided consumers with some degree of choice. Fundholders are also in a seemingly ideal position to act with knowledge and authority on behalf of their patients (Le Grand and Bartlett, 1993). However, the extent to which such choice is exercised in practice is unclear, and where it has been used it is again unclear whether the move is as a result of dissatisfaction with the GP as a *purchaser* (of secondary health care), or as a *provider* (of primary health care). There is in fact little empirical evidence to support the notion that there has been any significant change in the movement of patients between GPs since the 1991 reforms in the UK (Smee, 1995). Moreover, it is worth noting that this particular type of health care agent market is based on nonprice competition: patients do not pay GPs for their care. Funding is through general taxation, although GP budgets are partly set on the basis of referrals and hence patient numbers on their lists. Other countries, such as Germany, have had a tradition of health care agent competition based on the particular organisation of social insurance. However, as with fundholding in the UK, there is a great deal of inertia; most Germans tend to stick with their first choice of sickness fund. Such inertia can arise because the necessary effort, time and possibly cost needed to make choices may not be seen by consumers as worth the potential benefits they may gain by exercising choice. Perhaps one of the most undervalued benefits of universal health care systems is the lifting of the perceived burden of making choices (of doctor, of insurance scheme, etc.) particularly at those times (i.e. when ill) when most people are least able and willing to choose rationally. Freedom of choice – as with many other objectives in health care – is not the unalloyed benefit some would aver, but entails costs and trade-offs with other desired goals.

Whole market issues

Noted and alluded to throughout the foregoing discussion of supply and demand side issues has been the attempts by policy makers to wrestle with the problem that unconstrained markets in health care do not produce the full range of beneficial outcomes most often desired of such systems. Perhaps the key benefit of markets policy makers have tried to tap is the incentive system of markets based on the actions and behaviour of individuals rather than the state. So, for example, the choices made by individual consumers (choices of health care provider, or health agent, for example) are seen to better reflect individual health care needs (they are the best judges of their own welfare) as well as providing a powerful incentive for providers/agents to improve efficiency. In addition, markets can also serve a useful political purpose in seemingly distancing policy makers from difficult decisions about resource allocation or priority setting in health care. For example, within a command and control health care system, decisions about priorities are the responsibility of the state or its representative organisations. But experience of grappling openly with the complexity of the decisions and choices involved – from Oregon (Dixon and Walsh, 1991) to the Netherlands (Dekker, 1987) – suggest that governments do not want to be seen openly denying care and treatment to the populations they represent.

The problem with the use of markets as a solution to these problems is that other difficulties are created which require some form of ameliorating intervention. Perhaps the biggest policy hurdle to surmount is not the introduction of markets and market tools in health care, but the design of regulatory and market management processes which filter out the unwanted effects of markets without neutering their beneficial effects. Intervention by governments may actually increase rather than decline in this situation as they seek to grapple with these regulatory complexities.

Regulation, of what, how and by whom?

In the UK, as in a number of other countries, the privatisation of public utilities has spawned regulators charged with ensuring that newly divested industries do not exploit their position as natural monopolies. In certain cases the form privatisation has taken has, at least initially, reduced the degree of regulatory intervention by splitting up monopolies into smaller, competing firms. And, in the case of the UK at least, the role of the regulator was originally seen as a temporary interregnum between state and consumer sovereignty with competition eventually making regulation redundant (see, for example, Littlechild, 1985). However, in most cases, continuing regulation of one form or another has been seen not only as a necessary protection against monopoly, but as a way of ensuring certain desired outcomes which markets could not be guaranteed to produce even if markets developed towards some textbook perfection. In most privatised industries the role of regulation has in fact increased – perhaps beyond the level of state intervention inherent prior to privatisation (Helm, 1994).

Health care regulation, and market management in general, have been problematic, and many different forms have been employed to try to deal with the adverse effects of markets. For example, in the UK Acts of Parliament have limited the extent of markets. There is little or no competition between health agents, for example, and ultimate control of the system still rests with the Secretary of State for Health. In the USA a whole litany of three-letter acronymic market management policies have been tried over the years, from IPR to IPA HMOs. Approaches to regulation and market management clearly depend on the type, form and scope of the health care market; the extent to which competition is based on price or quality; where in the system (providers, health care agents etc.) competition or market tools are applied; the form of health care financing and the scope of other mechanisms (such as systems of arbitration to resolve trading disputes) employed to ameliorate market abuses.

Of course, the underlying guide for regulation must be the objectives of health care systems. But herein lie many of the difficulties of regulation or market management. The promotion of competition is often quoted as the objective of regulation, but competition is only a means to an end, not an end in itself (McGuire, 1996). However, all health care systems specify a range of goals, many of which are in conflict. Hence social value judgements are necessary on an almost continuous basis as to which goal should take priority over another in any given situation. Although regulatory rhetoric often specifies the pursuit of competitive rather than restrictive solutions to regulatory problems, the interpretation of this rhetoric in practice is often confused and inconsistent due to an inherent vagueness in defining the true purpose or end goals of regulation. So, for example, economies of scale associated with monopolies may be forgone in seeking a competitive solution to potential market exploitation of monopolists. Such trade-offs can be difficult to recognise, let alone quantify. But even when the true goals are properly specified, there is no guarantee that a regulatory process would necessarily always make the most socially beneficial decisions.

Conclusions

Two main questions underlie the thrust of this book: why has so much reform in health care been influenced by market ideology, and why now? In answering these questions it would seem most likely that there are a range of reasons for policy makers' current interest in markets, many of which are based on an underlying economic belief in the power of market mechanisms to provide a framework of incentives which encourage the greater pursuit of certain health care objectives (primarily technical efficiency).

But clearly, the choice of policy tool and the responsibility for implementation rests primarily in the political domain. Hence the distancing of politicians and the political process from difficult (potentially vote-losing?) decisions in health care cannot be ignored as an appealing characteristic of markets. The extent to which this has turned out to be the case in practice is debatable. Indeed, it is likely that the introduction of markets has heightened the link between politics/politicians and priority-setting decisions within health care in many countries. But perhaps two of the most important reasons for current trends in markets in health care has been previous experience with privatisation of public utilities and the inevitable pendulum swings in public policy.

Privatisation (arguably the ultimate use of markets in previous command and control systems) of state-owned, state-run firms provided, if not a model for change in health care, at least a dramatic change in the consensus about government ownership and running of industries. This, it could be argued, provided the political leap of faith required to consider how market mechanisms could be used to solve the perceived problems of health care systems. With privatisation it was no longer obvious why the state should, as Dieter Helm has noted, produce anything. Almost any activity could be contracted out to the private sector (Helm, 1994). But health care was and is different from telecommunications, gas, electricity, water and so on. Privatisation, or at least the use of market tools in health care, took on a different form not only within countries which had privatised other industries (i.e. most countries around the world), but between countries given their different starting points and the propensities for change in health care.

The inevitable pendulum swings in public policy making can also take some credit for the rash of market-based initiatives in health care. They are inevitable in the sense that rightly or wrongly, problems with health care systems, whether it be cost escalation, perceived technical inefficiencies, or whatever, will be associated with the dominant organisational form and economic framework existing at the time. In such circumstances, therefore, it is likely that solutions to problems will be cast in terms of opposite forms of organisation and economic frameworks. For command and control systems these will tend to be markets. In terms of the apparent pervasiveness of market solutions across many different countries, one simple explanation is the model of policy diffusion based on leader countries. For many states, the UK is considered such a leader, in privatisation and in health care. The NHS and subsequent policy changes in the UK's health care system since 1948 have provided many other countries with ideas and examples for developing their own health care systems. This does not imply slavish adherence to some health care policy path laid down by the UK, as clearly the UK does not have a monopoly (regulated or otherwise) on health care policy prescriptions. The situation is more complicated, with policy ideas flowing backwards and forwards across state boundaries. However, there are political benefits in being able to point to other countries as examples of potential ways forward in circumstances where unique political action can be seen as dangerous.

Finally, it is worth noting that the experience and use of markets and market tools has not been unique to health care. Even a cursory glance at other types of markets reveals the fact that no market exists separately or disconnected from the societal and political context in which it operates. All markets are shaped, regulated, managed and bounded by rules and conventions which, though they may change over time to reflect changes in societies' organisational and institutional structures and prevailing social values, nonetheless attempt to balance the benefits and costs of alternative methods of achieving a whole panoply of desired ends. However, even after half a decade of the use of markets and market tools in health care systems previously characterised as command and control, the evidence of any beneficial effect on key health care objectives is at best equivocal.

References

Appleby, J. (1995) *Testing the Market: A National Survey of Clinical Services Tendering by Purchasers*, Research Paper 18, Birmingham: National Association of Health Authorities and Trusts.

Appleby, J. (1996) 'The unfinished business for Mr Dorrell', *Parliamentary Brief*, 4: 62–3.

Appleby, J., Little, V., Ranade, W., Robinson, R. and Salter, J. (1991) *How Do We Measure Competition?*, Project Paper 2, Birmingham: National Association of Health Authorities and Trusts.

Ashton, T. and Press, D. (1997) 'Market concentration in secondary health services under a purchaser-provider split: The New Zealand experience', *Health Economics*, 6 (1): 43–56.

Baumol, W. J. (1982) 'Contestable markets: An uprising in the theory of industrial structure', *American Economic Review*, 72(1): 1–15.

Baumol, W. J., Panzer, J. C. and Willig, R. D. (1982) *Contestable Markets and the Theory of Industrial Structure*, San Diego, California: Harcourt Brace Jovanovich.

Butler, J. (1994) 'Origins and early development', in R. Robinson and J. Le Grand *Evaluating the NHS Reforms*, London: King's Fund Institute/Policy Journals.

Cullis, J. and Jones, P. J. (1992) *Public Finance and Public Choice: Analytical Perspectives*, London: McGraw-Hill.

Dekker, W. (1987) *Bereidheid tot Verandering*, Amsterdam: Commissie Structuur en Financiering Gezondheidszorg.

Dixon, J. and Walsh, H. G. (1991) 'Priority setting: Lessons from Oregon', *Lancet*, **337**: 891–4.

Enthoven, A. (1985) *Reflections on the Management of the National Health Service*, Occasional Papers 5, London: Nuffield Provincial Hospitals Trust.

Enthoven, A. (1994) 'On the ideal market structure for third-party purchasing of health care', *Social Science and Medicine*, **39**(10): 1413–24.

Evans, R. G. (1974) 'Supplier-induced demand: Some empirical evidence and implications', in M. Perlman (ed.) *The Economics of Health and Medical Care*, London: Macmillan.

Fuchs, V. (1974) *Who Shall Live?*, New York: Basic Books.

Helm, D. (1994) 'British utility regulation: Theory, practice and reform', *Oxford Review of Economic Policy*, **10**(3): 17–39.

Le Grand, J. and Bartlett, W. (1993) *Quasi-Markets and Social Policy*, London: Macmillan.

Littlechild, S. C. (1985) *Regulation of BT's Profitability*, London: HMSO.

Ludbrook, A. and Maynard, A. (1988) *The Funding of the National Health Service: What is the Problem and is Social Insurance the Answer?*, Discussion Paper 39, York: Centre for Health Economics, University of York.

Maxwell, R. J. (1988) 'Financing health care: Lessons from abroad', *British Medical Journal*, **296**:1423–6.

McGuire, A. (1996) 'Where do internal markets come from and can they work?', *Journal of Health Services Research and Policy*, **1**(1): 56–9.

McGuire, A., Henderson, J. and Mooney, G. (1992) *The Economics of Health Care: An Introductory Text*, London: Routledge.

Miller, R. A. (1982) 'The Herfindahl–Hirschman index as a market structure variable: An exposition for anti-trust practitioners', *Antitrust Bulletin*, **27**: 595–620.

Mishan, E. J. (1981) *Introduction to Normative Economics*, Oxford: Oxford University Press.

Organisation for Economic Cooperation and Development (1992) *The Reform of Health Care*, Paris: OECD.

Pareto, V. (1972) *Manual of Political Economy* (Eds: A. S. Schweir and A. N. Page, London: Macmillan.

Propper, C (1995) 'Economic regulation and the NHS internal market', in A. Harrison (ed.) *Health Care UK: 1994/5*, London: King's Fund Policy Institute.

Smee, C. (1995) 'Self-governing trusts and GP fundholders: The British experience', in R. B. Saltman and C. von Otter *Implementing Planned Markets in Health Care: Balancing Social and Economic Responsibility*, Milton Keynes: Open University Press.

Williamson, O. E. (1973) 'Markets and hierarchies: some elementary considerations', *American Economic Review*, **63**: 316–25.

CHAPTER 4

The procompetitive movement in American medical politics

THEODOR R. MARMOR

In the early 1970s the debates about American medicine began to shift in a number of ways. Claims of 'crisis' became commonplace as stagflation strained American public budgets, as medical care costs continued to escalate faster than general prices, and as the uninsured again received prominent attention. The language of dismay eclipsed the former celebratory rhetoric. For much of the period after the Second World War, American medicine experienced a golden age of expansion: in scientific research, in the growth of medical institutions, and in the vigorous efforts to distribute these gains more widely in reforms of the 1960s like Medicare, Medicaid, and the community mental health movement.

A sense of urgency marked the atmosphere of those medical care debates in the early 1970s, as political elites competed in designing remedies for a medical world that suddenly seemed too costly, too complex and too callous in an era of rapid inflation and with a growing number of uninsured.[1] While in the 1990s both American political parties try to distance themselves from any hint of 'big' government interventions, in the 1970s Republicans and Democrats, liberals and conservatives, actually competed over which form of national health insurance to offer in response to this widespread perception of distress in American medical care.[2] It is worth remembering as well that in the early 1970s it was assumed that the necessary tools of reform would be intensified governmental planning and more vigorous regulation of clinical quality, the costs of care, and capital investment. By the end of the 1970s, however, this reformist perspective had been discredited and debunked by many. To promarket critics, the answer was less regulation, not more, and competitive reforms became a dominant feature of policy debates about American medicine (see Marmor, 1990).

The rise of procompetitive ideas in American medical care: 1970–90

At least three factors made the increased attention to competitive ideas an understandable development. First, traditional concerns about access to medical care and the distribution of its costs began to take a back seat to worries about controlling the total cost of care. Problems of the uninsured and poorly protected could not compete for the public's attention with the genuinely ominous numbers on medical inflation. In 1970, the United States, possessing a strong and growing economy, spent 7.4 per cent of its GNP on health care (US Bureau of the Census, 1990:92). In 1980, with a weak economy still reeling from the twin oil shocks of the previous decade, the proportion was 9.1 per cent (*ibid.*). By 1991, medical care absorbed 11 per cent of the GNP (*New York Times*, 1991).

A second factor was the general ascendence, in academic writing, of a particular micro-economic approach to analysing public policy, or more accurately, as Melhado pointed out, the ascendance of economic analysis that had a deregulatory mission.[3] The anti government, free market enthusiasms of Milton Friedman's school of economists at the University of Chicago conventionally represent this development, but others who would hardly be associated with that movement, like Brookings economist Charles Schultze, were also influential (Melhado, 1988: 1–45). Indeed, it is fair to say that the neoclassical training of most American economists of this period made the growth of economic analyses of public policy a factor in this assumptive shift. All of this provided the intellectual groundwork for making procompetitive reforms more plausible in medical care. Indeed, Melhado cites a personal telephone conversation in which 'Alain Enthoven reports that he had read Schultze's book [*The Public Use of Private Interest*] shortly before devising his Consumer-Choice Health Plan and that he regards his [own] book as the "working out" in the health care economy of an example of Schultze's general propositions' (Melhado, 1988:87 n.65).

A third factor bolstering the so-called competitive movement was the spread of such antigovernment, antiregulatory sentiment to the wider political arena. Although this has become synonymous with Ronald Reagan, it in fact had earlier roots. Americans often forget the extent to which Jimmy Carter ran for president on an anti-Washington, antigovernment platform, portraying himself as a down-home farmer who, with pitchfork in hand, was headed to the nation's capital to slay the federal leviathan.

Three differing conceptions of procompetitive thought

The procompetitive ideology that arose out of the ashes of the 1970s had considerable political and rhetorical appeal. The simple version of the 'competitive' answer was that all social service delivery systems needed to be restructured to accommodate market incentives. In medical care, the most zealous proponents of competition predicted that a return to the market would lead to a more sensible control of costs, a more equitable allocation of scarce medical resources, the creation of a more rational delivery system, and the delivery of more appropriate (and perhaps better) medical care. The appeal of these procompetitive claims was broad enough that the *Report of President's Commission for a National Agenda for the Eighties* (1980), for example, could argue confidently that:

> An expansion of the role of competition, consumer choice, and market incentives rather than government control is more likely to create the much needed stimulus toward greater efficiency, cost consciousness, and responsiveness to consumer preferences so visibly lacking in our present arrangements for providing medical care.

Similar claims received widespread coverage in trade journals (see, for example, Christianson and McClure, 1979), the popular press, and on Capitol Hill (see Demkovich, 1980).[4]

The positions advanced under the label of procompetitive were, in fact, quite diverse and distinguishable. They varied in the degree of change proposed for American medicine, the rationale for such change, and their mechanisms, implementability, and effects. At the same time, while quite separable threads of procompetitive logic ran through these positions, there were some connections among the different proposals. Most importantly, the common ideological appeal to the wonders of markets and competition blurred the substantial differences among three conceptions.

The view that emerged first in the 1970s emphasised that patients should pay more of their medical bills and face the economic consequences of their consumption decisions. These advocates of 'consumer sovereignty' believed that the absence of significant patient cost sharing in health insurance was the major problem in American medical care. Near complete prepayment for care removes the necessity for both the consumer (patient) and the provider (doctor, hospital) to make trade-offs among different medical services and between medical care and other desired economic goods. Even if the consumer were not fully at risk for the cost of medical care, according to this line of argument, the use of deductibles, co-insurance, and co-payment would lead consumers to select more economically appropriate forms of care. In short, if the consumer is the best guide to what is desirable and affordable, medical care requires patients to pay.

The second competitive approach was more organisational in emphasis. It took for granted that American medicine provided too few acceptable alternatives to a fee-for-service payment and unorganised medical practices. Of course, medical competition had always existed within what came to be called fee-for-service (FFS) medicine. But it was not between conventional practice and other delivery and financing models like health maintenance organisations (HMOs), as they would have preferred. This organisational reform perspective encouraged the development of physician groups, primarily in prepaid group practices (PPGP), as an alternative to FFS medicine.

The proponents of the third view advocated aggressive antitrust rule making and litigation to reduce the market power of medical providers.

While the other reformers assumed the restructuring of financial systems and altering of reimbursement methods to allow competition on the basis of price, the advocates of antitrust had a somewhat different conception of the primary problem. They contended that collusive behaviour on the part of established medical providers prevented the emergence of competition in the market for medical care. Antitrust law, if enacted, would place a singular emphasis on the benefits of competition. The antitrust preference for competition above any other goal implied that any cost-containing effects of physician or medical system organisation would be rejected if the effects were brought about through a lack of competition or by the domination of the market by a particular group.

These were the three broad conceptions of procompetitive medicine and, as noted above, they were not necessarily independent of each other. Antitrust action could be used to eliminate barriers to the development of competing groups of medical professionals, a result compatible with the provider reorganisation approach. The cost-sharing approach might well permit indemnity insurance – with fee-for-service reimbursement – to compete with the insurance prices of prepaid group practice. These instrumental connections, however, were less important than the ideological commonalities to which the proponents appealed. All three procompetitive proposals rejected governmental regulation in the abstract and espoused 'correcting' the market they so admired. Procompetitive advocates carefully chose their label, in part to draw an explicit contrast with earlier reform approaches that relied on direct government provision of health insurance. The implication was that other reform proposals were anticompetitive and proregulation. Much of the intuitive appeal of procompetitive proposals was that they represented a form of autoregulation, the suggestion that the 'invisible hand' would sort out who got what without the heavy hand of public regulation and management. The fact that competitive plans all required extensive regulation to work never received the attention it deserved in this period.[5] And that in turn helps to explain why, over time, the disputes in American medicine pitted idealised models of market transactions with portrayals of actual governmental programmes, warts and all.

Market talk and medical care: the impact on the profession and the public

Not only was there a perceptible increase during the 1970s in the attention paid to proposals to make American medicine 'more competitive', but a dramatic shift simultaneously took place in the language of medical commentary. This transformation can be presented as a case study of what George Orwell might have called 'The politics of the medical language'. To change thinking, one manipulates language. The traditional doctor–patient relationship becomes, in competitive talk, provider–

consumer, or buyer–seller, or supplier–demander. Medicine becomes just another business. The fallout from this refashioned language came to be a threat to the professional ethos of American medicine.

Traditionally, much of the 'income' doctors, nurses and other medical practitioners earned has been noneconomic: self-esteem, respect from the community and idealisation as selfless professionals. In casting medical care as no different from other industries, medical professionals are reconceptualised. They no longer deserve (and increasingly no longer receive) the noneconomic benefits of public esteem, patient idealisation, and the gratitude of families. The stereotype of the medical professional as a self-interested (selfish) agent of business feeds on itself. And, over the quarter century we are surveying, the public's esteem for medical practitioners indeed fell sharply.[6]

Part of the decreased satisfaction with American medicine undoubtedly arose from worries over costs. Although it is impossible to establish a clear causal connection between the demystification of the medical profession and the increased costs of doctors, the phenomena have gone hand in hand. Despite sharp increases in the number of new physicians, doctors' incomes grew by 30 per cent from 1984 to 1989. (This contrasted with an average 16.3 per cent increase for other full-time workers over the same period (Fuchs, 1990).) Physicians' fees for procedures were approximately 234 per cent higher in the United States than in Canada (Fuchs and Hahn, 1990), and their take-home pay was more than 50 per cent higher than that received by Canadian doctors (Evans *et al.*, 1989). It should not be surprising that to the extent professional medical work was increasingly regarded as ordinary commercial activity, higher physician fees (and incomes) were increasingly understood as the result of market power or greed rather than a professional's just desserts.

Patient dissatisfaction begat doctor dissatisfaction. Despite the increase in incomes, the prestige of the medical profession decreased over the 1970s and 1980s. Doctors complained that they no longer enjoyed the autonomy they once had. Rather, elaborate and expensive procedures including utilisation reviews, requirements for pre-admission certification and other forms of second-guessing proliferated. AMA surveys in 1986, for example, found that 60 per cent of physicians strongly opposed third-party reviews of their hospitalisation decisions (Harvey, 1986). In an often-quoted 1991 article in *The Atlantic,* Regina Herzlinger reported that more than 30 per cent of current physicians said they would not have attended medical school had they known what their futures had in store (1991: 71).

The language of industrial economics and competitive markets did not just affect doctors. Hospitals and hospital administrators recast themselves in new terms. The hospital administrator increasingly became the chief executive officer. Assistant administrators were refashioned as vice-presidents for their respective functions. These changes were not merely semantic exercises. Rather, they represented a fateful change in the way Americans were encouraged to think of medical care. The vision of a hospital as primarily a business – and the concomitant shift in administrative power away from medical staff and toward professional managers – has inevitably affected the way Americans regard medical care. It would be wrong to assume unanimity on this and equally wrong to presume that American physicians and nurses think of themselves as simply business figures. The point here is narrower. Over time, the attack on the professional standing of medicine helped to deflate public confidence and to increase the probability of proposals threatening professional autonomy.

As hospital administrators gave way to chief executive officers (CEOs), so too did their incomes change. By 1990, hospital CEOs earned an average base salary of over $103,000; those receiving incentive pay averaged $125,000. Note that the salaries of these chief administrators increased by 8.5 per cent (on average) in 1989, while the Consumer Price Index grew by 4.6 per cent (Herzlinger, 1991: 74). And this took place in the midst of a supposed 'crisis' in health spending.

There are, of course, advantages to treating hospitals more like a typical business. Improved capital budgeting, financial and accounting systems are all vital in getting better value for health expenditures. Nor can one pretend medical practitioners are all selfless workers concerned only for the welfare of their patients. Clearly economic motives are important. Indeed, many of the concerns of those who subscribe to procompetitive strategies are identical to my own. Asymmetries of information and bargaining strength between doctors and patients require attention no matter what the context. Likewise, uncertainty about the efficacy of alternative treatments and the problems of moral hazard and adverse selection all need to be addressed whatever one's personal philosophy of entitlement to medical care.

But the rhetoric of the competitive reform helped to disguise what sets medicine apart from other industries and it was that broader development in part that made it possible for a Democratic president like Bill Clinton to marry ideas of universal health insurance to 'pro-market' ideology.

The robustness of market proposals

In arguing against government-financed or provided medical care, procompetitive advocates regularly claimed that governments are not sufficiently competent to manage such programmes. The inevitable concessions of the political process made sure, according to this line of argument, that programmes in action bear scant resemblance to their initial design. Over time, inefficiency sets in, as governments slowly respond to the results of their actions (which regularly include unintended consequences).

Ironically, as noted in the previous section, procompetitive advocates proposed a variety of detailed government programmes, laws and regulations designed to address and eliminate the market failures that occur in unregulated medical markets. The dilemma, hardly faced in most American public discussion of competition, arises precisely here. What happens to the logic of procompetitive proposals when government incompetence contaminates the efforts to reform medical markets? How desirable can a plan for 'managed competition' be when only half of its provisions get enacted and implemented, when insurance companies are not required to offer specific types of plans, when the government increases, rather than eliminates, the tax deductibility of medical insurance? What happens if experience rating is allowed (insurers can offer lower premiums to low risk groups) but the government sets up no provision for high risk groups who find it difficult to get insurance at all?

The answer is that most procompetitive plans were not robust in precisely this crucial respect. They would not perform well unless conditions were just right. By the very detailing of the government actions required to eliminate market failures, backers of procompetitive reform implicitly acknowledged that without these remedies, a competitive system does not work very well.

What happened to health care reform in the 1990s?

The characterisation of medical care as just another business also had implications for the way in which the potential for improvement from government intervention came to be judged. The dichotomy drawn between private competition and public regulation invoked free choice and well-functioning markets on the one hand, and the failed socialism of Europe on the other. But the dichotomy was, and is, artificial and misleading. The properties of the medical sector are such that regulation of some kind has always been regarded as inevitable by every serious writer on the subject. The most popular 'procompetitive' schemes, as noted earlier, all entail a myriad of restrictions on practitioners and patients alike.

It should be emphasised that what came to be called managed competition plans in the 1990s presumed the opposite of an unfettered market. On the contrary, these plans required extensive government regulation, as I have argued, regulation considerably more wide-ranging and complicated than that called for by more traditional universal health insurance plans. For example, in the competition between insurance plans encouraged by proponents of managed competition, some plans would have thrived by only attracting the young and healthy; while in rural areas, where it is often difficult to get a single medical provider to cover the population, competition among plans, whatever the encouragement, would have been totally infeasible. To avoid such imbalances, the architects of managed competition set up detailed rules to govern the system. These rules required all citizens to enrol through specified purchasing agents in one or another of a limited number of pre-approved plans. For their part, participating insurance companies were required to offer, not a single plan, but several predetermined varieties.

But it is not only managed competition that has to be managed. Despite a common procompetitive rhetoric, other reform proposals of the late 1980s and early 1990s presumed an extensive regulatory framework to combat market failures. (Indeed, the language of market failure provided the rationale for market reforms.) The plan proposed by the Bush administration, for example, explicitly prohibited health insurance firms from using experience rating in pricing their policies. The Heritage Foundation's proposal, to take another illustration, did not ban experience rating. Instead, it relied on state-regulated and administered insurance pools to cover high-risk individuals as an alternative instrument to deal with the same problem of unaffordable insurance prices for those with a history of illness.

The legacy of the two decades of debate over medical care reform between 1970 and 1990 was two-fold. On the one hand, the case for an American version of recognisable national health insurance – a Medicare programme for all, let's say – was weakened. Critics used the problems of American medicine to condemn governmental incapacity. On the other hand, promoters of competition in medicine compared idealised dream worlds with real systems (and, guess what, ideal systems seemed plausible). To persuade the public of the creditability of the idealised market world, the language of health debates was shrewdly altered. The vocabulary and terminology of economists became the vernacular, and the unquestioning use of this jargon became much more pervasive in debates.

It was in that context that Bill Clinton came to select managed competition within a global budget as his reform dream. That choice was fateful. It was doomed to political controversy for precisely the reasons we have stated. One has to regulate competition in medical care to make it acceptable, but if one does that and increases insurance coverage, the role of government is plain and the attackers have a field day.

The Clinton debacle and national politics

It all began so promisingly in the first months of the Clinton administration. When President Clinton introduced the issue of comprehensive health reform onto the national stage, support for fundamental reforms appeared enthusiastic and widespread. His presidential campaign had benefited from the remarkable reform consensus that had emerged over the 1980s: the idea that American medical care, particularly its financing and insurance coverage, needed a major overhaul. The critical unanimity on this point, what political sociologist Paul Starr rightly termed a 'negative consensus', bridged almost all the usual cleavages in American politics, between old and young, Democrats and

Republicans, management and labour, the well paid and the low paid. Americans had come to spend more on, and feel worse about, medical care than their economic competitors, with nine out of ten (including Fortune 500 executives) telling pollsters in 1989 that American medical care required substantial change.

Yet the speed with which the issue of comprehensive reform rose to the top of the public agenda was closely rivaled by the rapidity of its disappearance. The electoral reversal of November 1994 – the Republican takeover of both houses of Congress – underscored the Clinton administration's difficulties with health reform (and other issues). The Clinton administration had failed completely to persuade the United States Congress to enact health insurance reforms along the lines of 'managed competition', which raises the first explanatory question.

The demise of the plan in 1994 issued in a complex legacy. The period of political turbulence which followed proved a hospitable one for rapid, and often unprecedented, changes to the field of American medical care. In what is undoubtedly one of the great ironies of twentieth century American politics, the Clinton health reform debacle may also have removed the possibility of enacting major reform in health insurance from the political landscape.

In place of national health insurance, the Clinton reform effort has left a series of puzzles. Numerous explanations have been offered for the failure of the Clinton administration to carry out its comprehensive plan for reforming American medicine. Perhaps because what seems most striking, in retrospect, is the singularity of the strategy chosen and its unexpected consequences, most accounts have focused on specifics of the situation such as the complexity of the plan, the quality of leadership, the timing of political events and so forth.[7]

It has been argued, for example, that events beyond the control of the Clinton administration, such as the controversial passage of the North American Free Trade Agreement, the disastrous UN intervention in Somalia, or the ongoing dilemma of Bosnia, intervened at politically inopportune moments to draw the administration's (and the American public's) energy and attention away from the health care reform effort.

Others have emphasised the importance of both the internal and external timing of events. The external version is simply that the recession ended too soon, and with it, public concern about jobs, incomes, and employment-related health insurance. This undermined a key source of reform pressure. Moreover, this 'premature' recovery underpinned the Republican challenge to the need for comprehensive reform. On this view, the 'what crisis?' campaign by the Republican leadership cast doubt on the case for system overhaul at a critical juncture.

The internal version of the timing argument has to do with the policy development process itself. Although this argument has included many subthemes, the dominant version characterises the Clinton administration as having squandered its 'window of opportunity' by becoming mired in a complex and time-consuming development process. Careful

policy development of this sort may work against the chances of enact-
ment by giving opponents of the policy time to mobilise their consti-
tuencies and refine their rebuttals.

Finally, *The Health Security Act*, itself 1342 pages long, was arguably too complex and bureaucratically cumbersome to have any hope
of being understood, let alone embraced, by the general public. (A summary of the key proposals is given in Box 4.1).

Box 4.1 The Clinton administration's health care reform plan: key proposals

Coverage:
Guarantees health coverage for all American by 1998 by requiring
employers to pay at least 8 per cent of their employee's premiums
as of 1 January that year.

Scope of benefits:
Mandates a package of specific benefits covering routine doctor
visits, hospitalisation and emergency services, preventive care and
limited coverage for mental illness and substance abuse; prescription drugs; rehabilitation services; hospice, home health and extended nursing care services, and laboratory and diagnostic
services.

Form of administration:
Requires that states set up large consumer groups called 'health
alliances' to collect premiums, bargain with health plans and
handle payments. All companies with 5,000 or fewer employees
will have to get coverage through an alliance.

Financing:
Requires employers to pay at least 80 per cent of the average health
insurance plan in their areas for unmarried workers and an average
of 5 per cent of the family plan, but no more than 7.9 per cent of
payrolls for companies with fewer than 5,000 workers. Companies
with 75 or fewer employees and average wages of $24,000 or less
are eligible for subsidy.

Other:
Raises the current 24 cents/pack cigarette tax by 75 cents, to 99
cents. Limits the annual increase in the price of health insurance
premiums after the year 2000 to the rate of inflation, adjusted for
population and other socioeconomic factors.

Source: *Congressional Quarterly*, 10 September 1994, pp. 20–1.

The proposals tried to satisfy both those who would have preferred a single-payer model of national health insurance[8] with no role for the private insurance sector, and those who would have preferred nothing more than minor adjustments in rules governing health insurance. This strategy satisfied neither group and so, on this argument, was doomed to failure.

Although these narratives count as partial explanations for the failure of various movements for comprehensive health insurance in the United States, this frame of analysis focuses attention on solutions that respond to these supposedly circumstantial failures. Various remedies have been proposed. Appropriate planning, it has been suggested, required a more bipartisan and open process, one far less technocratic and closed than the Clinton task force. The press needed to take on a responsibility to educate, not merely to report, political food fights. What was called for – and will be again – is a simpler and more 'incremental' approach, one that genuinely respects current structures and avoids the fearful prospect of untried and uncertain ones (Morone, 1994; Yankelovich 1995; DiIulio *et al.*, 1994).

There is considerable optimism in all these remedial views. They presuppose that the goals of the Clinton plan were within reach. They take for granted that achieving guaranteed health insurance for all Americans, combined with effective cost constraints, requires only some shifts in the policy options proposed and the political tactics by which they are advanced. But this interpretation misses the real lesson of the Clinton administration's policy defeat in 1994. Though situational factors were undoubtedly implicated in the unfolding of events we have termed the Clinton debacle, they were not in themselves sufficiently important to account for the failure of the policy.[9]

The critical factors of demise

To understand the dismal fate of the Clinton administration's reform efforts, we must comprehend in a deeper way the constraints under which their ideological options and strategic choices were conceived and played out. This requires us to focus attention on structural features of the American polity, most importantly the constitutional ways in which authority and power are dispersed. Reforms of the scope the Clinton administration proposed would be difficult to enact under any circumstances and the setting of 1993–94 supplied no special reason to believe the ordinary constraints would be relaxed. An inhospitable combination of institutional structures, political culture and fiscal realities limited the capacity for large-scale policy reform in an area like medical care, and the weaknesses surrounding each factor were powerfully manipulated by vested interests during the Clinton administration's campaign. From this perspective, America's recent failure to enact universal health insurance was an expected outcome of these structural realities.

To make sense of the Clinton initiative, one must recall its origins and objectives. Two political imperatives justified the Clinton campaign's promise of reform and the White House's mounting a serious effort to deliver it. The first was the level of American medical spending (already 13 per cent of GNP in 1993), with the additional force of predictions that, unreformed, American medical care would cost 18 per cent of GDP by the turn of the century (Burner *et al.*, 1992). With the USA already out in front of the OECD pack (Schieber *et al.*, 1993), and the gap between it and the rest of its competitors getting larger, there was increasing concern about the economic consequences of these increasing 'outlays'. Additional resources going into medical care meant less competitive American goods and services, lower exchange rates and more expensive imports, or lower American worker wages (Reinhardt, 1989; US Congressional Budget Office, 1992). American medicine had become, or at least seemed to be, a burden on general economic growth and prosperity.

The second imperative was the growing insecurity of middle-class America about the adequacy and stability of their health insurance. At any given point in the early 1990s, approximately 15 per cent of the population were without health insurance coverage, with many more having inadequate coverage (Employee Benefits Research Institute, 1993). But that was, and is, a static and incomplete view of the predicament. Over any recent two-year period, as many as 50–60 million Americans will have been without health care coverage. It was those *with* coverage, who wanted some assurance that they would be able to keep it and that it would be there when they needed it, who represented the potent political force. As the cost of coverage rose, more and more employers were eliminating or modifying the options they offered to their employees, and the private insurance sector was becoming increasingly adept at risk selecting, and payment avoidance (Light, 1992). Not only could middle-class working families not be sure that their current coverage would still be there next year, or next week, but they could be relatively sure that, if they had any health problems, switching jobs was likely to be a costly venture (because insurance coverage is rarely, if ever, portable across carriers in the USA).

With these problems widely (if superficially) understood, the Clinton vision of reform expressed two key initial objectives: to control the costs of American medicine, and to assure health security (or guaranteed lifetime insurance coverage) for all Americans. The details of the Clinton strategy for achieving these objectives are now well known, and will not be repeated here. Of course, there has been no shortage of reasons proffered for the proposal's demise. As noted earlier, a wide variety of factors were implicated in the unravelling and defeat of the Clinton strategy. Yet very few contributed decisively to the result. In my view, a large part of the story of American exceptionalism arises from an inhospitable combination of institutional structures and political culture (Morone, 1992).

It is helpful in examining the various claims about the failure of the Clinton plan to ask whether the absence of a particular 'reason' would have meant a different outcome. In some cases, the answer seems relatively simple. For example, I believe that the external events, the policy itself and timing, were secondary, at best. If not these particular external events, there would have been others. The nature of politics is that one never has the luxury of focusing on only one thing, and it would be naive of anyone to believe that the Clinton reformers thought this would be possible or desirable.

As for the policy and the legislative process, despite its length and apparent complexity, one must recall that the details of the Clinton legislation were never meant for public consumption. The details of the American Social Security Act, or the Environmental Protection Act are no less complex – little more than the titles are understood by the public – yet they became law. More important by far was the failure to communicate the key features and to counter effectively the vested interests' clever use of the media.

To sustain the external timing argument, one would have to believe that, had the US remained in recession, the plan, or a modification, would have been passed into law. There is apparently no evidence that would support such a view. The internal timing arguments are equally difficult to support, requiring that quicker introduction, or introductions, as part of the budget bill, would have resulted in passage, in this case possible, but not likely.

It is unlikely because of the politics, media coverage and interest groups. It may be, however, that the greatest single impediment to the passage of health reform in the first Clinton term was the debilitating interplay through the media among those with vested interests: the public, and their elected politicians. Compulsory health insurance is everywhere an ideologically controversial proposal that involves enormous financial, symbolic and professional stakes. Rearranging how health insurance is provided significantly shifts the hands into which the money from medical expenditures flows. Any major reform proposal involves, by definition, an intent to change the distribution of costs and benefits. In medical care, change invariably involves diffuse benefits, and concentrated costs: a little better insurance coverage for a whole lot of people, at the expense of lost or reduced incomes for those involved in the health insurance business; more integrated patient care (and, perhaps, better patient outcomes) through managed care, at the expense of reduced pharmaceutical company revenues, fewer (and lower) specialist physician incomes, and fewer hospital-based incomes; less unnecessary defensive medicine and lower medical and legal costs, at the expense of the incomes of malpractice lawyers; and so on.

Those with a strong investment in the status quo have the most to lose in the event of successful reform, and hence have far more powerful incentives to get their case across than do those attempting to make the case for the effect of reform on the average American. And calamitous predictions of the effects of reform tend to cohere more closely with the sort of story that the editors of every daily newspaper or television news magazine encourage their staff to seek out, than do careful analyses or dull interviews with experts. Furthermore, the organised interests have at their disposal resources that far outstrip those available to (or likely to be committed to) a 'voice on the other side'. Not only do those interests represent important sources of campaign funding in an environment where election (and re-election) is prohibitively costly (Silver, 1995), but they are also able to support academics promoting 'friendly' proposals (*The Lancet*, 1993), and to engage high-priced and obviously quite effective help in the 'media influence' game.

Interest groups were particularly successful in manipulating two key beliefs which stand in the way of any health reform initiative that is likely to achieve cost control and universal coverage in the United States (Barer, 1995). The first of these is the firmly held belief that universal coverage will require additional revenue. The international evidence in fact provides striking proof that the opposite can be true. Because American medical arrangements were administratively inefficient and subject to demonstrably ineffective market or government restraints, a movement from private to public provision of health insurance might well have reduced the total share of GNP devoted to the nation's medical care sector. A second fundamental, perhaps even more deeply held, belief that stood as an impediment to 'successful' reform is the notion that the private sector more efficiently provides health insurance coverage than the public. To this day, and for obvious reasons, the private insurance firms continue to heavily promote this view. But that promotion is also given weight by many American health analysts who seem to believe fervently that private markets (the invisible guiding hand) must, by assumption, be able to respond to the preferences of a population far better than any government or public sector structures.

Of course, this view conveniently ignores the bulk of evidence to the contrary (Friedman, 1991; Light 1994). But it proceeds on the grounds that some additional private market reforms are all that stand between the current problems and health insurance nirvana. It is here that the optimistic view of market reform for market competition plays such an important role. Yet it seems obvious to most interested observers outside the United States that much of the activity in which the American private insurance sector engages is little more than waste motion, necessary only because of the peculiar ideological need (powerfully promoted, of course) to cling to the private market and support many corporate players. Risk pooling and community rating would eliminate the need for much of this 'busy work', but would, by definition, also eliminate many jobs and a lot of insurance company black ink.

Add to these the strong and enduring beliefs in the need to incorporate significant user fees in any reform package (presumably to control costs, but again in the face of compelling evidence to the contrary), and to hitch the funding of the system to place of employment (despite the complications and additional opposition from the business community so created), and one has a formidable set of structural impediments to any attempt at systematic medical reform. In the face of such a collection of strongly held beliefs, there seems to be little prospect of seeing either universal coverage or (even less likely) cost control in the United States in the near future.

In sum, it appears that politics, the media coverage, and organised interest groups, were the critical factors in undermining the Clinton effort at significant reform as well as any other option. But these are not separable elements, and it is their interaction that produced the mix of discourse to which the American public was subjected. By November 1994, the American public, which had earlier been so supportive of wide-ranging change, was now 'rejecting a major overhaul of the system' (Henry J. Kaiser Family Foundation, 1994:1). In the final analysis, disinformation and the spindoctors won out and the United States experienced another instance of public choice without policy change.

This time, however, the stalemated political outcome – symbolised by the literal disappearance of the Clinton plan in September of 1994 – was followed by an unprecedented pace of change in American medical care arrangements. Though this is not the place for any extended discussion, it is important for this assessment of the role of competitive medical care thought to note, in conclusion, whatever connections there have been between the long build up discussed earlier in the chapter and the Clinton debacle.

Conclusion

Over the years since 1970, there has been a constant and broad dispute over the proper role of government in capitalist democracies. The oil crisis of 1973–74 ushered in a period of stagflation that has only recently been transformed in the United States and has left a legacy of high unemployment throughout most of Western Europe.

In that context, the arguments in favour of increased competition – in medical care generally and particularly within health insurance – received far more favourable responses than at any other time in the period since the Second World War. There is, however, a crucial difference between Europe and the United States in this regard.

In Europe the argument for increased competition overwhelmingly took for granted that universal entitlement to health insurance was given, as other chapters in this book make plain. Not so in the United States. American arguments over the role of competition were part of the broader dispute over whether universal health insurance coverage was desirable and implementable. As a result, the story of this chapter is one of the rise of procompetitive ideas without a counterpart to the guarantee of insurance coverage.

The resulting story has been one of great hopes, great changes and great disappointment. The hopes of some of the procompetition advocates – of either the consumer sovereignty or organisational reform points of view – were a combination of universal coverage and competitive conditions in the pricing and delivery of medical care. The Clinton reformers also hoped to combine competition in the delivery of care with egalitarian financing of the basic insurance. Their hopes, as has been shown, were dashed completely, a tale of intellectual gullibility, naivety, and malleability that many American health policy analysts shared. Yet the story is more distressing than that. By capturing the interests and energies of so many reform actors, the procompetitive movement siphoned energy away from more appropriate strategies of reform in American public life.

The legacy of this rise and transformation of competitive ideas in United States medical care will be with America for decades. Without the regulation proposed by the Clinton plan, the advocates of so-called 'managed competition' have had a field day. The heady period – 1992–94 – was one of public choice debates without change. The period after has been one of tremendous change but without explicit choice. Some 70 per cent of Americans are now in insurance plans that are termed managed care. Most of those plans manage little else but costs, and, in doing so, restrict the choices of both medical professionals and their patients. In the name of expanding choice, American medicine has gone through a period of extraordinary reduction of choice. Aggregate health costs are rising at lower rates, but that is misleading. The ratio of medical care inflation to general inflation has not been markedly reduced. But the rise in costs to American firms has slowed, with the externalising of more costs – both fiscal and psychic – to patients and providers. Finally, there has been enormous change in the ownership and behaviour of insurers, hospitals, medical plans and drug firms. Consolidation describes much of what has transpired, with the growth of multihospital chains like Columbia HCA, the spread to nationwide activities of prepaid group practice organisations like Kaiser-Permanente, the spread of risk shifting through carving up capitation payments and having a galaxy of new firms manage less the medical services than constrain what care can be given and reduce or slow the rate of growth in the prices paid.

All of this constitutes an extraordinary set of ironies. In the name of competition, choice is narrowed. In the name of consumer responsiveness, consumer complaints have shifted in character and increased in anger. In the name of American entrepreneurialism, American physicians have been increasingly turned into employees of firms owned by others. Choice without change, change without choice, this captures the set of ironies but the working out will be in an America where national health insurance has been set aside as infeasible. The politics of medicine, as a result, will be increasingly fought out in state legislatures (see Rich and White, 1996). There the disputes will be over what degree of public regulation there should be over the enormous amount of private regulation that has already transpired. Very few observers would have predicted the subjects of controversy in the state legislatures of the mid-1990s: issues like drive-by mastectomies, limits of one day's hospitalisation for the delivery of a child or gag rules on what doctors could tell their patients about the limits of their managed care plans. Procompetitive enthusiasts did not predict such disputes either, but they have arisen in part because of the role of such ideas in the complicated politics of American medicine.

Notes

1. The realities of the fears were much exaggerated. For an examination of the hype see Marmor (1990).
2. In 1974, for instance, the now forgotten Kennedy–Mills proposal received extended consideration in finance committees of the Congress, as did the Nixon CHIP plan and the catastrophic health insurance bill of Senators Long and Ribicoff. To see just how broad this debate is, see de Kervasdoue *et al*. (1984: 234–57).
3. It may be hard to remember, but at one time economics helped to provide justification for government intervention and regulation: 'The principal motive for the increased application of economics to public policy after World War II was the expanding of government as a purveyor of large public programs entailing major expenditures (Melhado, 1988: 35).
4. All other industrial nations faced similar financial increases in medicine, yet the procompetitive vision of reform was uncommon to all but the United States. For a cross-national look, see Marmor *et al*., 1990).
5. Enthoven, for example, explicitly noted that competition required substantial regulation and strong management of the market in the DeVries Lectures of 1988. See Light (in press).
6. Public confidence in medicine and health institutions dropped from 73 to 33 per cent since the mid–1960s. While all major American institutions experienced a loss of public support, the medical profession lost support faster than any other professional group from the 1970s. Insofar as high levels of public trust are associated with altruistic behaviour and sense of social mission of a profession, at least some of the lost support was no doubt due to the increasing commercialisation in the medical profession. In his analysis of a host of survey data, Blendon found that while most (64 per cent of those polled) supported advertising by physicians, 58 per cent did not expect it to be truthful. For a more precise description of the poll, see Blendon (1988).
7. Here we are talking about the reasons for the failure of the Clinton plan after he made his choice. To understand the

conditions and history that led to Clinton's decision, see Hacker (1996, ch. 1).
8. A single-payer system is a universal coverage system under which the government collects funds for health insurance and has a uniform plan for everyone in a given state or nation. The arrangements effectively eliminate private health insurance for basic coverage. The single-payer option, under the Clinton plan, permitted a state to choose to make direct payments to medical providers with no intermediaries.
9. After President Clinton's re-election, a political amnesia has led many to forget how badly he fared in health care reform, which contributed to the Republican victory in the 1994 elections and the re-emergence of Clinton's 'problem-with-character' issue. Only the over-reaching of the Gingrich Republicans with their contract with America, the government shutdown and the buoyant economy transformed the story and boosted Clinton's reputation.

References

Barer, M.L. (1995) 'So near and yet so far: A Canadian perspective on US health reform', *Journal of Health Politics, Policy and Law*, **20** (2): 463–76.
Blendon, R. (1988) 'The public's view of the future of medical care', *Journal of the American Medical Association*, **259**: 3587–93.
Burner, S.T., Waldo, D.R. and McKusick, D.R. (1992) 'National health expenditure projections through 2030', *Health Care Financing Review*, **14** (1): 1–29.
Christianson, J.B. and McClure, W. (1979) 'Competition in the delivery of medical care', *New England Journal of Medicine*, **301**: 812.
de Kervasdoue, J., Kimberley, J.R. and Rodwin, V.G. (eds) (1984) *The End of an Illusion*, Berkeley, California: University of California Press.
Demkovich, L.E. (1980) 'Competition coming on', *National Journal*, **12**: 1152.
DiIulio, J.J. Jr., Kettl, D.F. and Nathan, R.P. (1994) 'Making health reform work: The view from the States', *Brookings Review*, **12** (3): 22(4).
Employee Benefits Research Institute (1993) 'Source of health insurance and characteristics of the uninsured', Issue Brief# 113, Washington, D.C.: EBRI.
Evans, R.G. *et al.* (1989) 'Controlling health expenditures – the Canadian reality', *New England Journal of Medicine*, **320**: 572.
Friedman, E. (1991) 'Insurers under fire', *Health Management Quarterly*, 3rd quarter: 23–7.
Fuchs, V.R. (1990) 'The health sector's share of the Gross National Product', *Science*, **247**: 534–7.
Fuchs, V.R. and Hahn, J.S. (1990) 'How does Canada do it?', *New England Journal of Medicine*, **323**: 886.
Hacker, J. (1996) *The Road to Nowhere*, Princeton, New Jersey: Princeton University Press.
Harvey, L. (1986) *AMA Surveys of Physician and Public Opinion: 1986*, Chicago: American Medical Association.
Henry, J. Kaiser Family Foundation (1994) 'News release', 1 November.
Herzlinger, R. (1991) 'Healthy competition', *The Atlantic*, **268**: 69–82.

The Lancet (1993) 'Editorial: US health reforms: clichés, cost and Mrs C', **341**: 7911–3.

Light, D.W. (1992) 'The practice and ethics of risk-related health insurance', *Journal of the American Medical Association*, **267**: 2503–8.

Light, D.W. (1994) 'Life, death, and the insurance companies', *New England Journal of Medicine*, **330** (7): 498–501.

Light, D.W. (in press) 'The economic sociology of managed competition', *Millbank Quarterly*, **75** (3).

Marmor, T. (1990) 'American health politics, 1970 to the present: Some comments', *Quarterly Review of Economics and Business*, **30**: 4.

Marmor, T., Mashaw, J. and Harvey, P. (1990) 'Crisis and the Welfare State', in T. Marmor, J. Mashaw and P. Harvey (eds) *America's Misunderstood Welfare State: Persistent Myths, Enduring Realities*, New York: Basic Books.

Melhado, E.M. (1988) 'Competition versus regulation in American health policy', in E.M. Melhado, W. Feinberg and H.M. Swartz (eds) *Money, Power, and Health Care*, Ann Arbor, Michigan: Health Administration Press.

Morone, J.A. (1992) 'The bias of American politics: rationing health care in a weak state', *University of Pennsylvania Law Review*, **140** (5): 1923–38.

Morone, J.A. (1994) 'The administration of health care reform', *Journal of Health Politics, Policy and Law*, **19** (1): 233–7.

New York Times (1991) 30 December: A10.

Reinhardt, U.E. (1989) 'Health care spending and American competitiveness', *Health Affairs*, **8** (4): 5–21.

Report of the President's Commission for a National Agenda for the Eighties 78–79 (1990).

Rich, R. and White, W.D. (1996) 'National health reform: Where do we go from here?' in R. Rich and W.D. White (eds) *Health Policy, Federalism and the American States*, Washington, D.C.: Urban Institute Press.

Schieber, G.J., Poullier, J.-P. and Greenwald, L.M. (1993) 'Health spending, delivery and outcomes in OECD countries', *Health Affairs*, **12** (2): 120–9.

Silver, G.A. (1995) 'Topics for our times: Clausewitz vs Sun Tzu – The art of health reform', *American Journal of Public Health*, **85** (3): 307–8.

US Bureau of the Census (1990) *Statistical Abstract of the United States, 1990*, Washington, D.C.: US Government Printing Office.

US Congressional Budget Office (CBO) (1992) *Economic Implications of Rising Health Care Costs*, Washington, D.C.: CBO.

Yankelovich, D. (1955) 'The debate that wasn't: The public and the Clinton health care plan', *Brookings Review*, **13** (3): 36 (6).

CHAPTER 5

Canada: markets at the margin

RAISA DEBER and PAT BARANEK

Health care in Canada

How much should society alleviate individual misfortunes? For decades, most industrial societies have accepted a public role for ensuring that everyone could receive medical care, without regard to their ability to pay. More recently, however, the welfare state has come under attack for reasons of both economics and ideology. As economic growth faltered, it was widely believed that governments no longer had the fiscal capacity to maintain existing levels of spending and service delivery. The globalisation of economies required countries to be internationally competitive and increased the pressure to harmonise social policies, to the extent that governments were becoming as accountable to international moneylenders as to their own electorates. At the same time, the rise of neoconservatism also suggested that governments no longer had the moral authority to interfere with the lives of the rugged individualists living within their boundaries. Winds of change thus began to sweep through most of the OECD countries. Canada was not immune. However, unlike many of the other nations considered in this volume, Canada to date has largely resisted market-based approaches for other than services at the margin (e.g. long-term care). Most of Canada's current reform activities have proceeded in other directions, often imposing even greater government regulatory control on the activities of providers and care recipients.

A brief description of the system

Medicare – the term commonly used to refer to universal hospital and medical care insurance in Canada – is among Canada's most popular programmes. An excellent account of its growth can be found in Taylor (1987); see also Deber (1993).

Medicare arose from an uneasy compromise between the public desire for uniform coverage for all Canadians, and constitutional and political limitations on the ability of the national government to act. Canada is a federation of 10 provinces (plus two thinly populated Northern territories), and national unity is a perennial concern (Tuohy, 1992). For decades, the country has been almost paralysed by the effort to reconcile the aspirations of the French-speaking province of Quebec with the views of the English-speaking majority in the 'rest of Canada'. As Cairns has noted, Canada has attempted to cope with three mutually incompatible views of the federal–provincial relationship (Cairns, 1991). If Canada is a partnership between French and English – a view often maintained by Quebec – Quebec should be entitled to half of the power. This position, which also leaves no role for aboriginal Canadians or the large multicultural population arising from massive immigration, is unacceptable to the rest of Canada. If Canada is an equal partnership among provinces – a view often maintained by Western Canada – Quebec would have one-tenth of the power. Unsurprisingly, this position is unacceptable to Quebec. Finally, if Canada is a partnership among all of its citizens, provincial power would be proportional to population. Under this position, Quebec would have about one-third of the power, with the likelihood that this would continue to diminish over time as population shifted westward. For some time, the resulting paralysis had been partially finessed through the device of devolving authority to the provincial level, so that matters of concern to Quebec would not be decided in the national arena. This escape hatch was modified in 1982 by the acrimonious passage – without Quebec's assent – of Canada's Constitution and Charter of Rights, which subjected Quebec policy directions to judicial review at the federal level. A series of subsequent attempts to deal with the issues arising have failed, revealing the extent of disagreement within the country, and leaving a legacy of acrimony, fatigue and ongoing uncertainty about national survival (Simpson, 1993). The election of a provincial government dedicated to taking Quebec out of Canada has heightened the stakes. Although Canada is already highly decentralised, current political trends accordingly encourage even greater devolution of powers to the provinces (Milne 1986; Olling and Westmacott, 1988).

Health care has been caught in the constitutional battles. Among the powers assigned exclusively to provincial legislatures by Section 92 of the *Constitution Act, 1867* were the provisions of section 92 (7) 'The Establishment, Maintenance, and Management of Hospitals, Asylums, Charities, and Eleemosynary Institutions in and for the Province, other than Marine Hospitals' (Government of Canada, 1982). Court decisions have interpreted this clause as assigning jurisdiction to provincial governments for almost all of the health care system; other powers assigned to the provincial level (e.g. education) have been interpreted as also giving the provinces jurisdiction over such matters as professional licensure. For the historical and cultural reasons noted above, constitutional roadblocks are not easily removed.

In theory, one would accordingly have to accept great discrepancies in availability of services in policy arenas under provincial jurisdiction. As shown in Table 5.1, Canada's 10 provinces, which range in population size from less than 130,000 to just under 11 million (that is, even the largest is smaller than the client base of many US insurance companies) vary considerably in their economic capacity. (Because the most recent data available on health spending is for 1994, we also present 1994 GDP data to preserve comparability.) Left to their own devices, the poorer provinces would clearly have less ability to sustain such social programmes as health care, even if they wished to do so. The table understates the economic disparities, because a significant part of the economy of the Atlantic provinces (Prince Edward Island, Newfoundland, Nova Scotia, New Brunswick) and almost all of the economy of the Northern territories (Yukon, Northwest Territories) consist of federal transfer payments which are being rapidly eroded as the federal government attempts to reduce its own deficit.

Table 5.1 **The population and GDP of Canada's provinces**

Province	Population[1]	GDP		
		Total[2]	Per capita	Relative (Canada = 100)
Nfld.	568,474	9,839	17,308	63
P.E.I.	129,765	2,418	18,634	68
N.S.	899,942	18,198	20,221	74
N.B.	723,900	15,089	20,844	76
Quebec	6,895,963	167,493	24,289	88
Ontario	10,084,885	303,151	30,060	109
Manitoba	1,091,942	25,041	22,933	84
Sask.	988,928	23,082	23,340	85
Alberta	2,545,553	83,182	32,677	119
B.C.	3,282,061	98,910	30,137	110
N.W.T.	57,649	2,165	37,555	137
Yukon	27,797	846	30,435	111
Canada	27,296,859	749,414	27,454	100

1 Population of Canada, 1991 Census. *Source*: Statistics Canada.
2 Gross domestic product 1994 at market prices, in million $ Canadian.
Source: Statistics Canada CANSIM matrices.

In the Canadian tradition of 'muddling through', the problems were papered over with money; it was deemed to be constitutionally permissible for the federal government to use the power of the purse to induce provinces to comply with national objectives, although neither level of government has chosen to obtain legal clarification as to the limits of this power. Accordingly, Canada has made extensive use of what is termed 'fiscal federalism' as a policy vehicle (Courchene *et al.*, 1985; Olling and Westmacott, 1988; Rachlis and Kushner, 1994), whereby resources were transferred from the richer provinces (primarily Ontario, British Columbia and Alberta) to the rest of the country. In consequence, during the economically prosperous period following the Second World War, the federal government in Ottawa was able to establish a series of cost-shared programmes, first for hospital insurance and then for medical insurance, under which funds would be provided to provincial plans as long as these complied with a series of conditions. These terms were reinforced and elaborated in the 1984 *Canada Health Act*; under its terms, provincial plans will receive full federal funding only if they comply with the five national standards:

1. Universality: all those eligible for coverage must be insured.
2. Accessibility: 'reasonable' access to insured services, without any co-payments or deductibles. The Act provides for dollar-for-dollar withholding of federal contributions for any such direct charges to patients, which proved a sufficient incentive to eliminate all user fees for insured physician and hospital services (Heiber and Deber, 1987).
3. Comprehensiveness: coverage must include 'all insured health services provided by hospitals, medical practitioners or dentists, and where the law of the province so permits, similar or additional services rendered by other health care practitioners'.
4. Portability: interprovincial arrangements must be put into place to ensure seamless coverage of insured people when they move from province to province.
5. Public administration: for efficiency purposes, the plan did not build in a profit margin for private administration of the insurance plans. (Canadian administrative expenses have been relatively low; to the extent that the US General Accounting Office estimated that the United States would be able to insure its entire population without additional costs if they could get American administrative expenses down to the Canadian level (United States General Accounting Office, 1991). However, recent efforts to improve the information available for management purposes have probably increased administrative expenses throughout Canada, particularly at the hospital and regional authority levels.)

These national conditions say nothing about how the plans should be managed; provinces can and do vary in how hospitals and physicians are organised and paid. Indeed, should any provincial government be willing to incur the fiscal penalties, it would also be free to violate any of the national standards. In addition, the terms of the Act establish obligations between governments only; there is no provision for individual redress. The 'Canadian' health care system is accordingly a series of provincially run insurance plans which reimburse private provision of what was seen to be a comprehensive array of services. The system was seen as a highly successful one, but has come under recent strains.

Limitations in what is publicly insured

One set of dilemmas arises from erosion of what is included within Medicare. The comprehensiveness definition was written relatively narrowly, based on an assumption that sickness was always managed in hospitals and by doctors. This assumption is increasingly obsolete; technology has allowed much care to be provided in community or home settings, and to be delivered by nonphysicians (Deber *et al.*, 1993; Deber *et al.* 1996). In effect, technological and organisational trends have led to creeping deinsurance, or what the Canadian Medical Association has termed 'passive privatisation' (Canadian Medical Association Working Group on Health System Financing in Canada, 1993).

Table 5.2 presents Health Canada data for the mix between public and private financing across sectors in 1992 (Health Canada, 1996), figures which probably underestimate private sector spending for nontraditional services (Deber and Swan, 1997). These figures nonetheless indicate that 74.1 per cent of health expenditures came from public sources (a figure which has been declining over the last few years), and that the public share varies considerably across sectors. At one extreme, the services included under the *Canada Health Act* definitions of comprehensiveness remain firmly within the scope of public financing: 91 per cent of hospital spending and 99 per cent of physician spending came from public sources. In contrast, the majority of spending on such rapidly growing categories as other health professionals, drugs (recognising that a considerable proportion of drug costs are hidden within the hospital budget), nursing homes and assistive devices come from private sources.

These figures cast some light upon the political implications of what is often referred to as 'rebalancing' the system. For decades, a series of examinations of provincial health care systems have concluded that the separation of provincial health care budgets into a series of 'silos' or 'stovepipes' (e.g. separation between budgets for hospital, physicians and community-based services) has led to irrational and suboptimal resource allocation (Newhouse, 1978; Angus, 1992; Mhatre and Deber, 1992). If one recomputes the data in Table 5.2, one recognises that the majority of public funding in 1992 went for hospitals (47 per cent), other institutions (9.5 per cent), and physicians (20 per cent), whereas the majority of private funding went for drugs (30.8 per cent) and other health professionals (27.3 per cent). (The private funding for institutions primarily reflects chronic care as well as surcharges for such noninsured extras as semiprivate or private rooms.) It is also noteworthy that the best cost control appears to have been precisely in the areas with the greatest proportion of public financing (Deber and Swan, 1997; Deber *et al.*, 1996). However, without reforms in funding arrangements, a shift to community-based care might in effect privatise such services, and hence would gain little support from either the public or providers.

Economic pressures

Reliance upon fiscal federalism worked as long as the federal government was willing to transfer 'enough' money to the provinces.

Table 5.2   **Health expenditures by subcategory of expenditure, 1992**

Subcategory	Public sector (million $)	Private Sector (million $)	Public %	Private %	Total (million $)
Hospitals	**24,369.1**	**2,408.9**	**91**	**9**	**26,788**
Other institutions	**4,944.2**	**1,889.9**	**72.3**	**27.7**	**6,834.1**
Physicians/psychologists	**10,368.7**	**95.2**	**99.1**	**0.9**	**10,463.9**
Other professionals	**965.6**	**4947.2**	**16.3**	**83.7**	**5,912.8**
of which:					
Dentists/denturists	326.8	4,269.8	7.1	92.9	4,596.6
Other professionals	638.8	677.4	48.5	51.5	1,316.2
of which					
Chiropractors	198.2	Not given			
Optometrists/orthoptists	205.6	Not given			
Podiatrists	18.7	Not given			
Osteopaths/naturopaths	2.4	Not given			
Private duty nurses	4.5	Not given			
Physiotherapists	209.4	Not given			
Drugs	**2862.6**	**5,589.0**	**33.9**	**66.1**	**8,451.6**
of which					
Drugs - prescribed	2862.6	3,187.5	47.3	52.7	6,050.1
Drugs - nonprescribed	0	1,122.7	0	100	1,122.7
Health personnel supplies	0	1,278.8	0	100	1,278.8
Capital	**1,721.4**	**557.1**	**75.5**	**24.5**	**2,278.5**
Other expenditures	**6,646.1**	**2,666.9**	**71.4**	**28.6**	**9,313**
of which					
Home care	915.6	Not given			
Ambulance	783.2	Not given			
Eyeglasses	18.1	1,295.3	1.4	98.6	1,313.4
Hearing aids	11.9	Not given			
Health appliances	294.0	Not given			
Unspecified services	216.9	Not given			
Prepayment administration	416.3	808.2	34	66	1,224.5
Public health	3,280.5	Not given			
Health research	463.8	264.2	63.7	36.3	728
Miscellaneous health care	245.8	Not given			
Other private health care	Not given	299.2			
All categories	**51,877.7**	**18,154.2**	**74.1**	**25.9**	**70,041.9**

Source: Health Canada (1996) *National Health Expenditures in Canada, 1975–94*, table 13A

Table 5.3   National health expenditures in Canada, 1994

	Total[1] Relative (Canada = 100)	Provincial[2] Relative (Canada = 100)	% of Prov. Expend. Programmes[3]	Total[4]	% of Provincial GDP Total[5]	Public Sector[6]
Nfld.	91	98	30.8	26	13.5	10.3
P.E.I.	93	89	27.6	23.5	12.7	8.7
N.S.	90	87	32	25.8	11.3	8.1
N.B.	96	97	32.3	26.7	12.1	8.6
Quebec	91	95	28.6	24.7	9.9	7.2
Ontario	105	104	35.9	30.7	9.5	6.6
Manitoba	103	95	32.8	25.6	11.5	8.3
Sask.	95	90	28.2	23	10.3	7.6
Alberta	97	95	31.5	27.2	7.9	5.9
B.C.	106	109	32.7	29.3	9.7	7.1
Canada	100	100	32.2	27.8	9.7	6.9

Source: Health *National Health Expenditures in Canada, 1975–94*
1. Computed from Table 15B. Total health expenditures (public and private sectors) in $ per capita, relative to Canadian total = $2,477.52
2. Computed from Table 17B. Provincial government health expenditures by province, excluding federal government direct, municipal government, and worker's compensation health expenditures, in $ per capita, relative to Canadian total = $1,642.47.
3. Table 31. Provincial government expenditures on health as a proportion of total programmes (total expenditures minus debt charges).
4. Table 32. Provincial government health expenditures as a proportion of total expenditures.
5. Table 27. Total health expenditures as a percentage of GDP by province.
6. Table 28. Public sector health expenditures as a percentage of GDP by province.

Similarly, providers were content to operate within government insurance plans as long as they received 'sufficient' resources from the province. Both of those assumptions fell victim to poor economic growth, coupled with the legacy of decades of deficit spending. Although most provinces and the federal government now spend less on programmes than they raise in revenues, the interest burden from previous debt has severely constrained the ability to act. Table 5.3 presents Health Canada data about health spending per capita, as a percentage of provincial budgets and as a percentage of provincial product. (Because so much of their revenues come from the federal government, the data for the thinly populated northern Yukon and Northwest Territories are not precisely comparable, and are accordingly omitted from all but the totals.)

Examination of health expenditures as a proportion of provincial/territorial GDP clarifies that these are already a greater burden to the poorer provinces. Whereas the Canadian average was 9.7 per cent, the lowest spending province in dollars per capita (Nova Scotia) nonetheless had devoted 11.3 per cent of GDP, whereas the highest spender

(BC) spent 9.7 per cent. The least burden on the provincial economy (7.9 per cent) occurred in the oil-producing western province of Alberta, and the highest (13.5 per cent) in the poor Atlantic province of Newfoundland.

As the result of several decades of deficit financing, by 1996, 35 per cent of the total revenue collected by the federal government had to be paid for interest on the national debt. Provincial governments were in danger of finding themselves in similar straits. For example, under the social democratic NDP provincial government, who decided to use fiscal stimulus to combat the recession, the province of Ontario ballooned their debt from $3.8 billion in 1990 to $97.5 billion five years later, the proportion of Ontario's revenues required to pay the interest exploding from 9.3 per cent to 17.8 per cent (Thorsell, 1996). One by one, governments have, enthusiastically or reluctantly, bit the bullet and turned to massive spending cuts. The federal government found immediate savings in curbing provincial transfers, unilaterally changing funding formulas, and removing billions of dollars expected by the provinces. In turn, with about one-third of provincial budgets devoted to health care, provinces found restraining health care spending an obvious target. The provinces have accordingly diverged; continuation of this trend is likely further to increase the gap among provinces in what they can afford, and even call into question the ability of the poorer to sustain existing programmes.

Political pressures, constitutional and ideological

Federal restraint in turn removed the primary mechanism of fiscal federalism. Without as much federal money, there was little to counterbalance the perennial cries from the provinces for massive decentralisation and an even more diminished federal role. These cries came primarily from the richer provinces of Western Canada (especially Alberta) as well as from Quebec. At the same time, the 1993 election saw the collapse of two of Canada's three national parties (the Progressive Conservatives and the NDP both reduced to too few seats to have official party status in the federal legislature), and left the ruling Liberals without a coherent opposition. The official opposition was the Quebec- based Bloc Québécois, which held no seats outside Quebec and concentrated primarily upon agitating for Quebec sovereignty. The Western-based Reform Party did not have enough support across the country to make it likely it could win a majority of seats. The Liberals were thus relatively free to reduce transfers to the provinces.

Coupled to the fiscal stringency was a rise in neoconservative ideology, much of which spilled across the US–Canadian border. Although there was little support for the radical views of the Gingrich Republicans, tough economic times made many Canadians less willing to support social spending. Federally, the Western-based Reform party argued for smaller government and tax cuts and spoke in favour of the growth of private medicine and the withdrawal of federal attempts to impose national standards in areas of provincial jurisdiction. Ideologically similar provincial Progressive Conservative parties won power in Alberta (under Ralph Klein) and Ontario (under Michael Harris), and immediately proceeded to implement their antispending, antigovernment, antitax platforms.

Framework for policy

Public and private in the context of financing, delivery and allocation

The Canadian reaction to constraint clarifies that the terms 'markets' and 'privatisation' do not always mean the same thing. Language can be used very differently in different locations. Many of the interventions referred to under 'market' rubrics are not really markets at all. In particular, clarity requires an understanding of the various dimensions of health systems. Although there are many ways of characterising health systems (Kleczkowski *et al.*, 1984; Roemer, 1984; Organisation for Economic Co-operation and Development, 1987, 1990, 1992, 1994; Pfaff, 1990; Abel-Smith, 1992, 1994; Adams *et al.*, 1992; Deber *et al.*, 1994; Frenk, 1994; Saltman, 1994), we have found it helpful to focus upon the following three dimensions: *financing* health systems, *delivery* of health services and *allocation* of resources to providers (Adams *et al.*, 1992; Deber *et al.*, 1995, 1996). The arguments about the appropriate public and private roles thus differ, depending upon which dimension of health services we are speaking about.

Those advocating a private role in financing have made their argument on a number of mutually contradictory grounds. (An excellent review of the issues is contained in a series of papers by Evans and colleagues (Evans *et al.* 1993, 1994; Stoddart *et al.*, 1993; Barer *et al.*, 1994; Bhatia *et al.*, 1994; Evans *et al.*, 1994a, b; Stoddart *et al.* 1994).)

The neoclassical economists argue that privatisation will reduce costs, bringing to bear the assumption that 'free' services will always be abused. As Appleby has also noted in this volume, the evidence instead suggests that a single-payer is the best way of controlling expenditures (Organisation for Economic Co-operation and Development, 1990; Deber *et al.*, 1996).

In contrast, providers argue that privatisation will bring additional resources into an 'underfunded' public sector. Implicit, but unstated, is that this approach will increase total costs. This view, although self-serving, is more clearly in accord with the evidence. However, although it is rational for providers to wish to evade cost controls, it is less clear why other members of society would be interested in paying more for health services without corresponding health benefits.

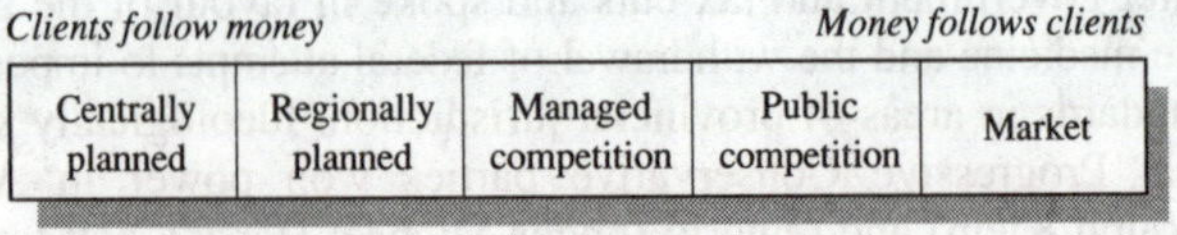

Clients follow money			Money follows clients	
Centrally planned	Regionally planned	Managed competition	Public competition	Market

Figure 5.1   **Allocation models for publicly financed services**

The third line of argument is less overt. One negative consequence of a single-payer system is that government has a conflict of interest between its dual roles as a payer and as the protector of the public interest. As anti-tax sentiment grows, there is a strong incentive for government to shift costs elsewhere, even if overall costs would be higher and equity would be impaired.

Although the same vocabulary is often used, clearly the policy aims sought by advocates of more competition in financing differ considerably. The political use of evidence is clear; the same policy proposals cannot simultaneously reduce and increase costs, and cost shifting is never overtly acknowledged.

Similarly, the arguments for a private role in delivery can have a number of bases. The primary line of argument has often rested in the critique of the state as provider. In general, there is strong agreement – often reflected in the 'reinventing government' movement (Osborne and Gaebler, 1992) – that replacing monopolies with competition in delivery is more likely to lead to client-sensitive services. These arguments also claim that competition is more likely to allow innovation. Others argue that allowing payers to 'shop around' among competing providers is important to force down costs (if one employs price competition), or to force up quality (if providers compete on those grounds).

The third dimension of health services in our framework is allocation – the mechanisms by which money flows from those who finance the system to those who deliver the services. Saltman and von Otter describe allocation mechanisms as lying along a continuum ranging from fully planned systems to pure neoclassical market systems (Saltman and von Otter, 1992). Figure 5.1 (above) shows our adaptation of their models.

The two most traditional means of allocating finances within health care systems are located at the extremes of the allocation continuum. *Centrally planned* allocation is associated with a command and control model in which the patient follows the money, that is, planners decide where particular services will be provided, and provide a global budget; patients must go wherever the services happen to be. Examples include the health system of the former Soviet Union, the National Health Service in Britain before the 1989 reform, or specialised hospital services in Canada. *Market* allocation, not to be confused with market-based financing, is a mechanism for allocating available resources (which may well be from public sources) to providers based upon the ability of providers to attract clients/patients, that is, the money follows the patients. Examples include physician services in Canada, as well as in the non-managed care portions of the United States system, that is, where physician income depends upon how many patients can be attracted. The clear advantage of the planned allocation models is cost control. The clear advantage of the market allocation mechanisms is increased sensitivity to patient choice, and therefore presumably to client needs and wishes.

The models found in the middle of the continuum represent various attempts to create a compromise between planning and markets which would ideally obtain the benefits of each without the corresponding flaws. It should be noted that most of these models are relatively new and untested. In many cases, they assign financial responsibility for delivering services to a particular group of identifiable patients for a range of identifiable services.

Managed competition models (which Saltman also refers to as mixed market models) create a mixed public/private market in which existing and new privately capitalised providers can bid for contracts against present publicly capitalised facilities. The central agent for change in this model is the administrative agent managing the health plan, who is responsible for overseeing service contracts to providers. Managers are expected to balance questions of quality and cost in the search for less expensive forms of care. The extent of patient choice is reduced to the selection of an administrative agent, who then makes choices on patients' behalf. If dissatisfied, their main option is to switch to another plan. In contrast, the models towards the market allocation end of the continuum tend to allow patients/clients to determine resource allocation (e.g. the public competition models described by Saltman, in which individuals choose which providers they will use, but total budgets can be capped (Saltman and von Otter, 1992, 1995)). With regional models, command and control is devolved to a regional body to which individuals are assigned on the basis of residence.

From this perspective, one can view allocation issues as being at the heart of the debate under way in many countries about separating the functions of purchasing and delivery (often referred to as the 'purchaser–provider split'). It is important to recognise that the concept of a split between purchaser and provider can apply only under one of the following conditions:

1. The third-party payers have disappeared, leaving the patient as the sole purchaser of services. This implies relinquishing the insurance model, and forgoing protection against catastrophic risks.
2. Decisions about where to receive services are no longer made by patients, but by a purchasing agent. The importance of patient choice as a value within the Canadian system may be one reason why such approaches have not as yet been widely adopted.

It is important to note that all of these allocation models operate within a framework of public financing. Many of the key issues can be related to the four basic policy goals as described by Stone (1988): equity (e.g. access), security (e.g. quality, comprehensiveness, implementation of a broader definition of health), efficiency (e.g. incentive structures, reduction of excess capacity, encouragement of integration and coordination, provider accountability) and liberty (e.g. the extent of consumer sovereignty, physician autonomy). Others, however, deal with the highly political concerns of power shifting (among providers, and among providers–payers–patients–managers etc.). Inevitably, in a time of attempted cut-backs, strategies can also focus on shifting the blame for reductions in services, access, and/or provider incomes.

Context for reform

The road to reform. Rise and fall of the ideology

Canada has relied upon public (single-payer) financing for those services covered by the *Canada Health Act*, coupled with private delivery (mainly not-for-profit, in the case of institutions, and small business, in the case of fee-for-service physicians). Public delivery has played only a very limited role (e.g. provincial psychiatric hospitals in some provinces), and there appears to be general agreement from all except affected staff about the appropriateness of government continuing to offload ('privatise') such direct service delivery. Ontario and Alberta, which have elected neoconservative governments, required government departments to prepare 'business plans'; those written by the health departments note an explicit intention to shift the role of government away from direct service delivery. More intensive use is being made of contracting out of services in an attempt to reduce their costs (often, by substituting lower cost nonunion labour for unionised hospital or government employees). Such competition is particularly prevalent for services which are not directly chosen by patients (e.g. the movement towards contracting out hospital services such as laundry or food service), or those not required to be insured under the *Canada Health Act*. As one recent example, the Capital Health Authority, which has responsibility for ensuring delivery of a wide range of health services in Edmonton, has cut funding for physiotherapy services by 30 per cent, and shifted to a 'preferred provider network'. Only 17 of the 56 private clinics in the region received contracts. However, the policy also left an 'escape hatch' for those who lost the competition to deliver services; at the same time, a new system of assessing needs was implemented, which would disqualify those with 'low needs' from publicly financed treatment. Presumably, those clients and clinics will form an alternative private market outside of the publicly funded system (S. Lowry, personal communication, 1995).

However popular their antitax rhetoric, neoconservatives have none-theless discovered that there is little public support for privatising health care financing. The existing system is very popular among the Canadian public (Blendon and Taylor, 1989; Blendon *et al.*, 1990); 'threats to Medicare' are a perennial election issue, and the public strongly op-poses 'two-tier medicine'. Canada thus provides an example of the dog which did not bark in the night: the most noteworthy development has been the absence of a major challenge to the principles of public financ-ing of medically necessary services coupled with private delivery. The primary reform activities instead relate to allocation policy, the link be-tween financing and delivery. This is not so much a public/private issue as an issue of degree of government control and the sorts of incentives built into reimbursement policies.

This support for the status quo, however, is more fragile than might appear at first glance. It has become evident that public support for comprehensive universal insurance is dependent upon maintenance of an implicit social contract that people can obtain high quality care in a timely manner within the publicly funded system. The growth of con-sumerist views further expands the public sense of what Medicare should cover. This increase in demand, it must be noted, is often cata-lysed by providers. Canada is near the USA, and influenced by US media. For example, pharmaceutical companies may advertise on tele-vision that, through the marvels of research, they have now helped re-solve a problem (often, one not previously considered medical, such as baldness). 'Ask your doctor', the ad concludes, thus generating new ex-pectations and new office visits. Articles in the popular press can lead to similar surges in demand. This expansion in demand soon collided with the desire of governments to restrain health care spending, and their eventual fear that they could no longer afford to provide comprehensive high quality care to all. The public reaction to attempts by governments to restrain funding, however, made it clear that individuals would not forego wanted care merely to preserve the public system. Faced with a clinician who told them that they 'needed' an MRI, for which there was a six-month waiting list, many were willing to pay extra to bypass the queue.

As noted in a background paper for the National Forum on Health (Deber *et al.*, 1996), a number of issues arise from offering preferential access to 'paying customers'. First, such clients are usually highly sub-sidised by the public system. Costing is rarely complete, and charges are often based on the marginal cost of adding an additional patient rather than upon the full expenses of maintaining the service (including training). In addition, the private clients often incur costs to the public system (labs, follow-up visits, etc.), including the medical costs of any resulting complications. This can be particularly problematic for risky or experimental procedures (e.g. stomach stapling); the Consumers' As-sociation of Canada (Alberta) (Consumers' Association of Canada, 1994) has estimated that the hidden costs of such services include the additional malpractice premiums which must be paid by all physicians.

Most crucially, there is a high risk that a private alternative will pull away resources and impoverish the publicly insured services. For example, physicians may choose to spend more time for private patients, allowing waiting lists for 'free' care to grow. A study of access to cataract surgery by the Consumers' Association of Canada (Alberta) found that the waiting list for patients whose ophthalmologists performed surgery only in the public sector was an average of two to six weeks. Longer waiting periods of up to 18 months for 'free' surgery were encountered only by patients of ophthalmologists with a dual practice; payment of an additional 'facility fee' to the provider would decrease the wait to about two to four weeks. However, in one clinic, if a referring physician had performed the necessary tests, surgery could be performed on the same day as the initial clinic assessment. These results suggest that the 'waiting list' issue pointed to by advocates of private clinics may in part be artifactual, since the lists appear to arise only if a second tier is permitted.

Acceptance of a private second tier, however, raises a number of questions. What mechanisms exist to moderate the inherent conflict of interest of clinics claiming that procedures are 'needed' in order to increase revenues? The well-known variation in surgical rates across jurisdictions leads to some concern, especially if there are incentives to overservice. Although there is no way to determine the 'correct' rate, the rate of cataract surgeries for residents of Alberta – where the renowned private Gimbel eye clinic is situated – is considerably higher than the rate in other provinces. The extent to which such clinics meet unmet demand, as opposed to helping to generate it, is therefore unclear. Another key issue is whether the existence of a privately financed alternative will allow the public sector to 'offload', assigning fewer resources to such care, and creating a self-fulfilling prophecy of 'shortages'. The USA again provides a cautionary example: 25 per cent of physicians simply refuse to treat Medicaid patients, while two-thirds of the remainder limit the number they will treat. Accordingly, patients in the US 'public' tier may not have access to willing care providers (Watson, 1995). The use of privately financed clinics has often been justified in terms that, in our view, apply only to public delivery (i.e. that such clinics are more innovative). This line of argument leads to confusion; there is no reason why such clinics cannot exist within the publicly financed system, should government decide that they are of sufficiently high priority. In the background paper for the National Forum on Health (Deber *et al.*, 1996), we argued that if there are indeed shortages of medically required services, the response presumably should be to reallocate resources. If resources to deliver medically necessary services are still inadequate (which seems unlikely given the current levels of health spending in Canada), it would appear preferable to raise that money through the public sector, rather than pay the increased costs (in diminished ability to control spending, decreased equity and increased burden on employers) which often accompany competition among financers. In addition, from a political standpoint, support for the public system is likely to erode if people perceive that they can obtain 'better' care outside of the current system (Deber *et al.*, 1996).

Medicare has worked to date because of the balance between what the system would provide, and what people thought they needed. The trends noted above have tended to disrupt the balance. First, the economy has led governments to believe that they can no longer afford to provide a first class system to all. Second, consumerism has led people to expect services beyond the level which can easily be justified as a compelling national priority, particularly if such expenditures are at the expense of other policy arenas (e.g. education, economic development) with higher paybacks in increasing the health of the population (Evans *et al.* 1994).

How will this dilemma be dealt with? Government cutbacks in effect break the implicit contract. The result is an urge to allow people to buy their way out. The past few years have seen a challenge to the nonprofit ethos, and a number of attempted 'quick fixes'. A popular one is to redefine comprehensiveness, and split coverage into 'core' vs. 'noncore' services (Canadian Medical Association 1994a, 1994b). Operationalising this, needless to say, has proven almost impossible, especially since the usual issue is not whether or not to fund a procedure, but for whom, and under what circumstances (Deber, 1992).

Most Canadian provinces have reacted to the economic pressures noted above by instituting some variant of regional reforms; these are examples of what Saltman terms adaptive planning and represent a shift towards the planned end of the allocation continuum. This would seem to indicate the dominance of cost control goals, as opposed to service quality and/or consumer responsiveness. As will be noted below, there have also been limited and selective use of market instruments, but primarily in sectors (e.g. long-term care reform) which are not included under the definition of 'comprehensiveness' and hence not subject to federal policy control.

The reforms: regionalisation, cost cutting and cost shifting

The key 'reform' direction has accordingly been setting up regional bodies and dissolving the boards of local hospitals and community agencies. The resulting districts tend to be very small (as small as 12,000 people in some Saskatchewan regions) and are not likely to be actuarily stable should plans to shift to a 'needs-based funding approach' be fully implemented. The stated rationale is to encourage a more balanced distribution of resources and break down the 'silos' between hospital care and community-based services. More cynical observers note that this strategy also 'diffuses the blame' for funding cuts. The regional bodies are often required to pull large sums of money away from hospitals; population-based approaches also mean that resources may be diverted from the larger cities. At the same time, small rural hospitals have also been closed. There has been minimal evaluation of the impact of these activities. Despite lip service towards 'community responsiveness', both providers and recipients of care appear to have lost power. One provincial government has already been defeated, largely due to opposition to 'health reform', and others facing imminent elections have accordingly been promising to move more resources into health care.

In an effort to retain service levels with diminished budgets, providers have incentives to downsize and deprofessionalise. Many nurses are being replaced by generic workers. Hospitals may cap budgets for beneficial procedures with high marginal costs, such as hip replacements, even though there are waiting lists. Although under strain, hospitals appear to be managing to continue to give the same level of service. The situation with physicians, however, is far more volatile. No province has as yet incorporated physician services into regional global budgets, and most physicians are still in solo practice fee-for-service practice, with the extensive overhead expenses implied by that mode of delivering health care services. Instead, provinces have relied on a variety of mechanisms for 'capping' the total budget to be paid to physicians (Lomas *et al.*, 1989). One approach was to retain fee-for-service, but implement 'clawbacks' on all physician billings if total billings exceeded an agreed amount. This formula created a 'tragedy of the commons' (Hardin, 1968), since those providers wishing to achieve a 'target income' had an incentive to increase their workload, and there were no mechanisms to ensure that resources went to needed services. Accordingly, those who ran 'revolving door practices' were rewarded at the expense of their more restrained colleagues.

In Ontario, fiscal pressure and the failure of physicians to come up with their own proposal for meaningful reform meant that by 1996, clawbacks had grown to over 10 per cent of physician billings, often imposing significant financial losses. The Conservative provincial government also introduced and passed the controversial omnibus Bill 26, which gave the government new powers to close and merge hospitals, force physicians to practise where the government felt they were needed, and not pay for 'unneeded' services or providers. Evidently believing that they could employ 'divide and conquer' techniques, the government also removed the Ontario Medical Association as the designated bargaining agent for physicians, as well as reneging on previous agreements (e.g. to help pay physicians' malpractice premiums). The predictable result has been escalating conflict between the province and the physicians. As of this writing, physicians have been working to rule and refusing to see new patients; in response, the province has threatened to use its new power to dictate where physicians can practise (Toughill, 1996). Although the ultimate resolution is unclear, the breakdown of trust does not bode well for the orderly restructuring of health

Table 5.4 **Alberta health budget**

	1992–3	1993–4	1994–5	1995–6	1996–7	Cumulative change (from 1992–3)
Spending (billion $)	4.166	4.03	3.824	3.659	3.694	
Change (million $)	—	–136	–206	–165	35	–472
% change from previous year		–3.3	–5.1	–4.3	1.8	–11.3

care to insure that it continues to provide high quality, timely, comprehensive care to all.

The attempt to restructure has been made both more pressing and more difficult by efforts to remove resources. The cuts – as opposed to merely lower rates of increase – began in the western province of Alberta, which has traditionally had an individualistic political culture. After his election in 1992, Alberta Premier Ralph Klein brought about an aggressive regionalisation programme which also involved cutting more than $470 million from a $4.16 billion budget over three years (see Table 5.4). Rural regions were relatively spared, while the Capital Health Authority (serving the city of Edmonton, which had not supported the governing party) was scheduled to take a funding cut of $176.6 million over that period. The measures required significant losses of personnel and closures of facilities.

Following Alberta's example, the Ontario government has started to remove over $1.3 billion from hospital spending, in effect erasing a decade of growth with no allowance for population increases or inflation. A cut of 5 per cent has already been implemented for 1996–7; with a 6 per cent cut scheduled for 1997–8, and another 7 per cent for 1998–9. This is proceeding in tandem with an effort to restructure Ontario's hospitals and close many of them; however, concerns have been expressed that the cuts are proceeding too quickly (often well before the restructuring commission's recommendations are given, so that hospitals do not know what services they will be responsible for).

The Ontario government is at the beginning of its mandate, and resistant to criticism. In Alberta, however, the resulting care deficiencies have resulted in a public uproar, with Mr Klein's government, facing an upcoming election, having found it advisable not only to rescind planned cuts, but also to restore total funding to near the preslash level. Public opinion polls continue to find strong public opposition to 'two tier medicine' and the erosion of Medicare.

Privatisation by attrition

In consequence, privatisation has been proceeding by stealth. There is anecdotal evidence that budgetary constraints are leading to problems with quality of care and timeliness; however true, they have evoked considerable concern among Canadians. The extent to which waiting lists are a real problem is not clear; neither is the extent to which Canadians are seeking care in the USA. Certainly, providers are trying to use these anecdotes to justify allowing a private second tier.

One interesting example of an attempt to destroy Medicare camouflaged in the language of support is the platform of the Reform Party. Their policy on Health Care, as obtained from the Reform Party website on 31 October 1996, includes:

A. The Reform Party supports the value of Medicare in providing essential, comprehensive national health services, publicly funded, portable across Canada and universally accessible to all Canadians regardless of financial status.
B. The Reform Party supports defining Medicare's essential services in consultation with users, health care professionals, the provinces and the Federal Government. Non-essential services would not be reimbursed by Medicare.
C. The Reform Party supports Canadians' freedom to access essential and non-essential health care services, beyond Medicare, if they so choose.
D. The Reform Party supports converting federal cash transfers to the provinces for health into additional 'tax points', which would provide a stable and growing revenue source for longer term provincial funding of Medicare.
E. The Reform Party supports the complete rearrangement of the concept of health care insurance, such as: basic deductibles, medisave accounts, choice of insurance coverage, and complete coverage for catastrophic illness.

Within the language of choice, the alert reader can detect the abandonment of any federal role in enforcing national standards (since 'tax points' cannot be withheld once granted); the end of any requirement to have comprehensive high quality services available within Medicare (both since 'essential' may fall far short of 'medically necessary', and since people could buy their way out of the system), the explicit identification of medical care as a commodity which people should be able to 'access' whether they need it or not, and the abandonment of a single-payer. The platform also begs the issue of provider influence on demand, assuming that the decision to 'access' a service is entirely consumer-driven.

An interesting question for future investigation may be the extent to which this move towards consumerism has also led to a gradual abandonment of reliance in trust in providers as a way of assuring quality, as well as to the erosion of the professional status of the medical profession.

Towards vertically integrated systems and primary care reform

Canadians have certainly been observing market-oriented reforms. There is a lot of talk about primary care reform: switching to capitated group practices (with considerable variation as to which costs should be included within the budgets, and the roles of physicians vs. other providers). There has also been interest in vertically integrated systems which would receive monthly payments for their rostered population, from which they would purchase (or provide) an identified range of services. These models include a semimoribund effort at developing comprehensive health organisations (Lamb *et al.*, 1991) and the current interest in integrated delivery systems (Leatt *et al.*, 1996). To date, this has produced conferences, papers and proposals, but not much action. In particular, there has been little attention to how one merges universal publicly financed coverage with 'choice' of organisation. Instead, it has been assumed that risk selection can be dealt with through adjusting the payment. Integrated competitive models are clearly inappropriate for most of Canada, since they assume a large enough population base to allow competing providers, and as such are most widely discussed in major urban areas (e.g. Toronto). In contrast, most provinces, as noted, have moved towards regional models which also attempt to integrate services, but give no choice as to which organisational entity will take responsibility for which population.

Long-term care reform in Ontario

Nonetheless, there is one clear example where market approaches are indeed going to be used, the most recent of over a decade of attempts to reform long-term care (LTC) in Ontario. We view LTC as a possible harbinger of longer term changes in other sectors, since it is not constrained by the requirements of the Canada Health Act. In the new model, the provincial government will allocate fixed budgets to organisations called community care access centres (CCACs). In turn, for-profit and not-for-profit private providers will have to compete for contracts with the CCACs. The differences between this reform attempt and the efforts of previous governments provides an instructive look at the importance of ideology in structuring reform.

For the most part, LTC services in Ontario had been provided through a 'patchwork quilt' of mostly unintegrated and unregulated services, offered through a jumble of for-profit, charitable, volunteer and municipal agencies on widely varying terms and conditions. In this pluralist heaven, no one agency had the mandate or resources necessary to monitor and coordinate services on an ongoing basis. While producing diverse services and programmes, this nonsystem posed significant problems of accessibility and equity to consumers. The absence of information and 'process barriers' created by fragmentation, inadequate coordination and different eligibility criteria resulted in many consumers falling through the net and not being able to find or access appropriate services. One consequence was felt to be an overly high rate of early or unnecessary institutionalisation as compared with selected other OECD nations. It was widely recognised that more appropriate placements should be able to relieve the pressure on acute hospital services, which in turn would require more availability of home support services.

Another consequence of the status quo was that consumers often faced a baffling task of trying to navigate through available services, which may have carried different costs and standards of care for purportedly equivalent services. Within a given sector of care, the responsible government ministry, legislation, funding policies, patient eligibility criteria and copayment formulas could vary. Pressure from interest groups to address these issues led to a growing belief within the government that the existing system was no longer sustainable. Successive Ontario governments accordingly attempted to reform long-term care services (Deber and Williams, 1995).

A series of proposals then ensued. They differed with respect to several key issues.

In terms of financing the issues were: what services would be included in a publicly funded programme? How much would be paid by government? By service recipients? Where would user charges be employed? Would government subsidisation be based on capitated formulas for a population, or on some other assessment of 'need'? Which client groups would be included? The frail elderly? The disabled? Those discharged from hospitals on the assumption that home care services would be available? In general, the models tended to concentrate on the frail elderly and the goal of avoiding institutionalisation, with the other potential client groups often being served by the same programmes having less of a say in the proposed models.

In terms of delivery, the issues were: would the reform be restricted to institutions and medically based home care services (e.g. nursing, physiotherapy, etc.)? Or would it begin to take in the vast array of social support programmes? What would be the role of public delivery? Not-for-profit private delivery? For-profit private delivery? Volunteers?

In terms of allocation: how would resources be allocated? Would there be competition for clients, or would a planned model (e.g. regional) be used?

Over the next 10 years, a series of models were proposed by three governments, which ran the gamut of potential government involvement. The initial proposal of the Liberal government in 1985 was for a very minimal government role as the provider of information, under what was called the 'one stop shopping' concept. Individuals would still decide which services they wished to receive, and from whom. It was soon substituted by a proposal for a more activist government role as a 'broker' and coordinator. The Liberals changed lead ministries and proposed to set up service access organisations (SAOs) which would act as a single access point to the system, combining information, referral, service coordination and service provision on a case-managed basis. This brokerage model was attacked as adding another layer of bureaucracy, but was well on the way to implementation when the Liberals lost the 1990 election.

Following renewed community consultations, the new NDP (social democratic) government initially proposed a similar model, which they renamed service coordination agencies (SCA). Following yet more consultations, however, the NDP shifted to a model which, in effect, adopted public delivery. The multi-service agency (MSA) also took a broader definition of health, and was intended to provide not only professional services (e.g. nursing, physiotherapy, etc.), but also a vast array of social support services currently being provided (if at all) by volunteer-based community agencies. The MSA budget was divided into categories to protect the social services and ensure that professional services would not absorb more than their 'share' of the budget. No MSA would be allowed to use more than 20 per cent of any budget category to purchase services, probably dooming the existing provider organisations. Instead, designated services would be provided by employees of the MSAs. The model evoked enormous controversy (including questions about the role of unions, the fate of volunteer workers and the ability to provide even the current extent of services within the new model). Before it could be implemented, the NDP lost the provincial election, and was replaced by a neoconservative Progressive Conservative government, which promised to scrap the MSAs.

In January 1996, the new Ontario Health Minister announced the latest attempt at reform: to streamline the 74 existing home care and placement coordination programmes into 43 community care access centres (CCACs). The CCACs were to purchase services from community providers; the press release returned to the language of 'simplified access'. Unlike the earlier brokerage models, the CCACs would provide no services themselves. The new model also returned to a more narrow definition of the services to be included under long-term care reform; it now included only professional care (nursing, physiotherapy, etc.), a limited range of community supports (Alzheimer day programmes), homemakers and admission to long-term care facilities, omitting the host of volunteer-based community supports (e.g. Meals on Wheels, transport, friendly visiting, security checks), which had been a key element of the MSAs.

The process for developing each of the reform models under the three different governments varied in terms of its openness, paralleling Paul Starr's lay definitions of public and private as open versus closed (Starr, 1989). At one extreme of the public/private continuum, the NDP government had held massive province-wide meetings, claiming to have consulted 75,000 individuals and groups. They widened the scope of conflict by funding the creation of new consumer groups made up largely of the healthy elderly who supported their vision for reform.

Voice was given to labour, consumer and volunteer provider groups, at the expense of professional provider groups.

When the Progressive Conservative party took over the government in 1995, they embarked on a rapid, small-scale, by invitation only consultation. The scope of conflict was narrowed, and influence shifted away from labour and consumer groups to provider groups, especially the for-profit sector who could be relied upon to support a competition model based on best price (particularly if there were no requirements for a unionised workforce, and few explicit ways of measuring quality).

Tracing the reform proposals makes the role of ideology clear. Because LTC is characterised by a large, diffuse and marginally resourced network of societal groups and the relative absence of constraints (e.g. nonapplicability of the Canada Health Act), it is easier for the successive reforms to be state-dominated and mirror each government's view of the appropriate role of government. Possibly because the Liberal party is seen as largely non-ideological, the Liberal models did not provide a major challenge to the existing system. However, the MSA model proposed by the social democrats of the NDP increased the role of government from one of partially financing services to include delivery; under their model, multiservice agencies would provide all designated services, with strong preference to be given to unionised workers over nonunionised workers. The private sector was directly disadvantaged by the limitation to 20 per cent of the MSA budget for the purchase of their services. This model accordingly threatened both the existing not-for-profit and the for-profit private sectors, who viewed it as 'expropriation without compensation'. Other client groups would also be affected. Some non-profit groups serving a varied client population feared that their organisations would not be able to survive without the budget arising from their provision of LTC services. Volunteer agencies believed that the new 'faceless, nameless bureaucracy' would not be able to attract volunteers, and therefore would end up costing the government more. Charities were unenthusiastic about providing funds to what were seen as government agencies, implying a decrease in available resources. For-profit agencies resented the explicit preference for the not-for-profit sector. The only groups who viewed themselves as winners were unionised labour and the relatively healthy elderly, who believed they would receive a broader array of social supports.

The MSA model was at the left-hand end of the allocation continuum, that is, central command and control, where client followed money. Although on the surface MSAs looked to be arm's length not-for-profit agencies, the legislation gave full power to the provincial minister of health not only to designate (or undesignate) MSAs, but to micromanage their activities, including approving the budget, imposing specific terms and conditions (including the choice of premises), to take over their powers, and to remove some or all of their directors. By mandating the services an MSA must provide, and by delivering those services, this model removed the choice inherent in the previous system. In shifting control over admission to LTC institutions from that institution to the MSA, the model enhanced 'equity' among individuals judged to have equal need for a given level of care, at the expense of 'equity' in being able to respond to ethnospecific or spiritually sensitive services.

The Progressive Conservative government adheres to a neoconservative ideology with a strong preference for reliance on the private sector. Accordingly, its CCAC model shifts the government's role back to partial financer, with the introduction of a purchaser–provider split in the allocation and delivery dimensions. Professional, homemaking and personal support services will be purchased by the CCACs on a competitive contract basis. Consumer choice will now be limited to influencing boards of directors of CCACs on their choice of agencies with which they will contract, or by purchasing nonpublicly funded services directly from the private sector. While the MSA model squeezed out the for-profit and non-unionised agencies, and the CCAC model will squeeze out the volunteer and not-for-profit groups, the capped budgets of both will allow governments to shift the burden of illness and ageing slowly and stealthily onto families and informal care givers.

Under the CCACs, for-profit and not-for-profit agencies will have to compete on the basis of quality and price for contracts. While the evaluation of quality is yet to be defined (some suggestions include client and staff satisfaction surveys), it seems that, in the meantime, price will be the determining factor. Recognising that the not-for-profit sector may be disadvantaged, the government has partially protected the funding of all agencies financed under the old home care program for a transitional period of up to three years in order to give them time to become competitive with the for-profit sector. Thereafter, the not-for-profit and the for-profits will have to compete on an even playing field, including competing with out-of-country agencies (largely US for-profit firms) who are currently poised at the border. The emphasis on competitive price is likely to result in the replacement of unionised workers with lower paid workers, and the replacement of professional providers with less qualified ones. Quality is likely to suffer. Agencies which are unsuccessful in obtaining CCAC contracts will have to rely completely on the private market (privately purchased insurance plans or out-of-pocket payments by consumers) for their continued existence. Privatisation by attrition is likely to occur. However, since LTC was not firmly established as part of the publicly funded system, the policy will be played out as a series of private dilemmas for individuals and their families. As accountability for care provision becomes more decentralised, there are fewer mechanisms for amplifying discontent.

Conclusions

To date, markets have stayed on the margin of Canadian health care. However, language is not always used the same way. In particular, there has been considerable confusion between a private role in financing, and in delivery. The consumerist debate, framed in the language of entitlements, further blurs the picture. A desire to have high quality 'client-focused' care implies attention to delivery and allocation mechanisms; it is too often worded in terms of eliminating single-payer financing, particularly by those wishing to evade cost controls.

In turn, the desire of governments faced with economic pressures and ideological propensities to favour the private sector have led to destabilisation of the existing bargain. Providers had agreed to operate within a single-payer system in the expectation that they would receive 'adequate' funds. Cutbacks in turn transform politics into a zero sum game, in which one can gain only if others lose. This in turn is slowly affecting the structure of interests in health care. Providers are losing ground to budget cutters. In turn, the culture within health care institutions is changing. This chapter did not deal with the likely undermining of trust and professionalism, the rise of the new managerialism, and the changing roles of doctors and nurses. Beyond the economists' issues of dollars and markets, however, rests a very fragile culture. At its core, health care is about taking care of sick people and preventing healthy people from becoming ill. To do so, it relies upon a vast array of expertise which few individuals can master. Ideally, health care is a partnership between patient and provider (Deber, 1994a, 1994b). Without trust, such a partnership is impossible.

Will LTC become a model for other parts of the system? Will markets emerge from the margin? Should they?

In the language of our framework, we believe that judicious use of market mechanisms of allocation can often be an important way of ensuring client sensitivity, assuming that adequate quality can be defined, measured and ensured. However, competition also implies sufficient excess capacity, and may be detrimental where populations are too small to support multiple providers, as well as where there are high barriers to entry. For example, how can one have competition for open-heart surgery unless you have units working under capacity? Is this desirable, both because of the relationships between higher volumes and improved outcomes, and because of the waste involved? In contrast, it seems very feasible to have competition for food services or housekeeping. Accordingly, delivery mechanisms will have to balance competition and co-operation. In the financing arena, however, we believe the evidence against 'markets' is overwhelming. Multiple payers are likely to make it more difficult to control total costs, and impair equity (including introducing problems of risk selection and adverse selection). However, retaining the single-payer system is likely to be difficult over the near future.

In our view, the battle over national standards remains crucial. Without a mechanism for identifying privatisation by attrition, erosion is likely. In turn, failure to maintain the explicit social contract to preserve universal access to high quality, timely, and comprehensive medically required services may indeed lead to greater support for the ability to obtain such care outside the publicly funded system. Policies like those suggested in the Reform Party platform, if adopted, may indeed signal the beginning of a slow decline in Canadian Medicare. The main protection is a vigilant population, and careful attention to the successes and failures of other countries which have experimented with markets as to their likely benefits and failures. If the canary in the mine shaft sings with a foreign accent, health services researchers may make their greatest contributions as translators.

References

Abel-Smith, B. (1992) *Cost Containment and New Priorities in Health Care*, Aldershot: Avebury Books.

Abel-Smith, B. (1994) *The Escalation of Health Care Costs: How Did We Get There?* High-Level Conference on Health Care Reform, OECD, Paris November 17–18.

Adams, O., Curry, L. and Deber, R. B. (1992) *Public and Private Health Care Financing: Literature Review and Description*, Volumes 1 & 2 (Addendum of Data Tables), Ottawa: Curry Adams & Associates.

Angus, D. E. (1992) 'A great Canadian prescription: Take two commissioned studies and call me in the morning', in R. B. Deber and G. G. Thompson (eds) *Restructuring Canada's Health Services System: How Do We Get There From Here?*, Toronto: University of Toronto Press.

Barer, M. L., Bhatia, V., Stoddart, G. L. and Evans, R. G. (1994) *The Remarkable Tenacity of User Charges: A Concise History of the Participation, Positions, and Rationales of Canadian Interest Groups in the Debate Over 'Direct Patient Participation' in Health Care Financing*, Toronto: Ontario Premier's Council on Health, Well-Being and Social Justice.

Bhatia, V., Stoddart, G. L., Barer, M. L. and Evans, R. G. (1994) *User Charges in Health Care: A Bibliography*, Toronto: Ontario Premier's Council on Health, Well-Being and Social Justice.

Blendon, R. J., Leitman, R., Morrison, I. and Donelan, K. (1990) 'Satisfaction with health systems in ten nations', *Health Affairs*, **9**(2): 185–92.

Blendon, R. J. and Taylor, H. (1989) 'Views on health care: Public opinion in three nations', *Health Affairs*, **8**(2): 149-57.

Cairns, A. C. (1991) 'Constitutional change and the three equalities', in R. L. Watts and D. M. Brown (eds) *Options for a New Canada*, Toronto: University of Toronto Press.

Canadian Medical Association (1994a) *Core and Comprehensive Health Care Services: A Framework for Decision-Making*, Ottawa: Canadian Medical Association.

Canadian Medical Association (1994b) *Core and Comprehensive Health Care Services: The Legal Issues*, Ottawa: Canadian Medical Association.

Canadian Medical Association Working Group on Health System Financing in Canada (1993) *Toward a New Consensus on Health Care Financing in Canada*. Discussion paper prepared by the Working Group on Health System Financing in Canada, Ottawa: Canadian Medical Association.

Consumers' Association of Canada (1994) *Current Access to Cataract Surgery in Alberta*, Alberta: Consumers' Association of Canada, Alberta Branch.

98 *Markets and Health Care: A comparative analysis*

Courchene, T. J., Conklin, D. W. and Cook, G. C. A. (1985) *Ottawa and the Provinces: The Distribution of Money and Power*, Volumes 1–2, Toronto: University of Toronto Press.

Deber, R. B. (1992) 'Translating technology assessment into policy: Conceptual issues and tough choices', *International Journal of Technology Assessment in Health Care*, **8** (1): 131-7.

Deber, R. B. (1993) 'Canadian medicare: Can it work in the United States? Will it survive in Canada?', *American Journal of Law and Medicine*, **19** (1 & 2): 75–93.

Deber, R. B. (1994a) 'The patient–physician partnership: Changing roles, and the desire for information', *Canadian Medical Association Journal*, **151** (2): 171-6.

Deber, R. B. (1994b) 'The patient–physician partnership: Decision making, problem solving, and the desire to participate', *Canadian Medical Association Journal*, **151** (4): 423–7.

Deber, R. B., Adams, O. and Curry, L. (1994) 'International healthcare systems: Models of financing and reimbursement', in J. A. Boan (ed.) *Proceedings of the Fifth Canadian Conference on Health Economics*, Regina: Canadian Plains Research Center.

Deber, R. B., Narine, L., Baranek, P., *et al.* (1996) *The Public–Private Mix in Health Care*, Ottawa: Report to the National Health Forum.

Deber, R. B., Ross, E. and Catz, M. (1993) *Comprehensiveness in Health Care*, Ottawa: HEAL, The Health Action Lobby.

Deber, R. B. and Swan, W.R. (1997) 'Puzzling issue 4: The public private mix in Canada', in M. J. Hollander (ed.) *Report on Five Puzzling Issues, and Fact Sheets, on Canadian Health Services in an international context*. A Report prepared for the National Forum on Health, Victoria: Canadian Policy Research Networks.

Deber, R. B. and Williams, A. P. (1995) 'Policy, payment and participation: Long-term care reform in Ontario', *Canadian Journal on Aging*, **14** (2): 294–318.

Deber, R. B., Williams, A. P., Baranek, P. and Duvalko, K. (1995) *Report to the Task Force on the Funding and Delivery of Medical Care in Ontario: The Public–Private Mix in Health Care*. Task Force on the Funding and Delivery of Medical Care in Ontario, Toronto: Government of Ontario.

Evans, R. G., Barer, M. L. and Marmor, T. R. (1994) *Why are Some People Healthy and Others Not: The Determinants of Health of Populations*, New York: Walter de Gruyter Inc.

Evans, R. G., Barer, M. L. and Stoddart, G. L. (1993) 'The truth about user fees', *Policy Options* **14** (8): 4–9.

Evans, R. G., Barer, M. L. and Stoddart, G. L. (1994) *Charging Peter to Pay Paul: Accounting for the Financial Effects of User Charges*, Toronto: Ontario Premier's Council on Health, Well-Being and Social Justice.

Evans, R. G., Barer, M. L., Stoddart, G. L. and Bhatia, V. (1994a) *Who Are the Zombie Masters, and What Do They Want?*, Toronto: Ontario Premier's Council on Health, Well-Being and Social Justice.

Evans, R. G., Barer, M. L., Stoddart, G. L. and Bhatia, V. (1994b) *It's Not the Money, It's the Principle: Why User Charges for Some Services and Not Others?*, Toronto: Ontario Premier's Council on Health, Well-Being and Social Justice.

Frenk, J. (1994) 'Dimensions of health system reform', *Health Policy*, **27**: 19–34.

Government of Canada (1982) *The Constitution Act, 1867*, Ottawa: Government of Canada.

Hardin, G. (1968) 'The tragedy of the commons', *Science*, **162**: 1243–8.

Health Canada (1996) *National Health Expenditures in Canada 1975-1994, Full Report*, Ottawa: Health Canada, Policy and Consultation Branch.

Heiber, S. and Deber, R. B. (1987) 'Banning extra-billing in Canada: Just what the doctor didn't order', *Canadian Public Policy*, **13** (1): 62–74.

Kleczkowski, B. M., Roemer, M. I. and Van Der Werff, A. (1984) *National Health Systems and Their Reorientation Towards Health for All – Guidance for Policy Making*, Public Health Papers #77, Geneva: World Health Organization.

Lamb, M., Deber, R. B., Naylor, C. D. and Hastings, J. E. F. (1991) *Managed Care in Canada: The Toronto Hospital's Proposed Comprehensive Health Organization*, Ottawa: Canadian Hospital Association Press.

Leatt, P., Pink, G. and Naylor, C. D. (1996) 'Integrated delivery systems: Has their time come in Canada?', *Canadian Medical Association Journal*, **154** (6): 803–9.

Lomas, J., Fooks, C., Rice, T. H. and Labelle, R. J. (1989) 'Paying physicians in Canada: Minding our Ps and Qs', *Health Affairs*, **8** (1): 80–102.

Mhatre, S. L. and Deber, R. B. (1992) 'From equal access to health care to equitable access to health: A review of Canadian provincial health commissions and reports', *International Journal of Health Services*, **22** (4): 645–68.

Milne, D. (1986) *Tug of War: Ottawa and the Provinces under Trudeau and Mulroney*, Toronto: James Lorimer.

Newhouse, J. P. (1978) *The Economics of Medical Care: A Policy Perspective*, Reading, Massachusetts: Addison-Wesley.

Olling, R. D. and Westmacott, M. W. (1988) *Perspectives on Canadian Federalism*, Scarborough, Ontario: Prentice- Hall Canada.

Organisation for Economic Co-operation and Development (1987) *Financing and Delivering Health Care: A Comparative Analysis of OECD Countries*, Paris: OECD.

Organisation for Economic Co-operation and Development (1990) *Health Care Systems in Transition: The Search for Efficiency*, Paris: OECD.

Organisation for Economic Co-operation and Development (1992) *The Reform of Health Care: A Comparative Analysis of Seven OECD Countries*, Paris: OECD.

Organisation for Economic Co-operation and Development (1994) *The Reform of Health Care Systems: A Review of Seventeen OECD Countries*, Paris: OECD.

Osborne, D. E. and Gaebler, T. (1992) *Reinventing Government: How the Entrepreneurial Spirit is Transforming the Public Sector*, Reading, Massachusetts: Addison-Wesley.

Pfaff, M. (1990) 'Differences in health care spending across countries: Statistical evidence', *Journal of Health Politics, Policy and Law*, **15** (1): 1–67.

Rachlis, M. and Kushner, C. (1994) *Strong Medicine: How to Save Canada's Health Care System*, Toronto: Harper Collins.

Roemer, M. I. (1984) 'The public/private mix of health sector financing: international implications', *Public Health Reviews*, **12** (2): 119-30.

Saltman, R. B. (1994) 'A conceptual overview of recent health care reforms', *European Journal of Public Health*, **4**: 287–93.

Saltman, R. B. and von Otter, C. (1992) *Planned Markets and Public Competition: Strategic Reform in Northern European Health Systems*, Philadelphia: Open University Press.

Saltman, R. B. and von Otter, C. (1995) *Implementing Planned Markets in Health Care: Balancing Social and Economic Responsibility*, Buckingham: Open University Press.

Simpson, J. (1993) *Faultlines: Struggling for a Canadian Vision*, Toronto: Harper Collins.

Starr, P. (1989) 'The meaning of privatization' in S. B. Kamerman and A. J. Kahn (eds) *Privatization and the Welfare State*, Princeton, New Jersey, Princeton University Press.

Stoddart, G. L., Barer, M. L. and Evans, R. G. (1994) *User Charges, Snares and Delusions: Another Look at the Literature*, Toronto: Ontario Premier's Council on Health, Well-Being and Social Justice.

Stoddart, G. L., Barer, M. L., Evans, R. G. and Bhatia, V. (1993) *Why Not User Charges? The Real Issues*. A discussion paper, Toronto: The Premier's Council on Health, Well-Being and Social Justice.

Stone, D. A. (1988) *Policy Paradox and Political Reason*, Glenview, Illinois: Harper Collins.

Taylor, M. G. (1987) *Health Insurance and Canadian Public Policy. The Seven Decisions that Created the Canadian Health Insurance System and their Outcomes*, Kingston, Ontario: McGill-Queen's University Press.

Thorsell, W. (1996) Blessed are the deficit-cutters for theirs is the Kingdom of Heaven', *Toronto Globe and Mail*, D8, Saturday, 26 October 1996.

Toughill, K. (1996) 'Tories' options on doctors range from capitulation to all-out war', *Toronto Star*, B5, 2 November 1996.

Tuohy, C. J. (1992) *Policy and Politics in Canada: Institutionalized Ambivalence*, Philadelphia: Temple University Press.

United States General Accounting Office (1991) *Canadian Health Insurance: Lessons for the United States*, Report to the Chairman, Committee on Government Operations, House of Representatives, Washington, D.C.: GAO.

Watson, S. D. (1995) 'Medicaid physician participation: Patients, poverty, and physician self-interest', *American Journal of Law and Medicine*, **21** (2–3): 191–220.

Acknowledgements

We thank our colleague A. Paul Williams for helpful discussions. This work was supported in part by Grant #6006-5583-302 from Health Canada, National Health Research and Development Program. We have also drawn upon work done by our team for the National Forum on Health and for the Task Force on the Funding and Delivery of Health Care in Ontario. We thank Ann Pendleton and Florinda Cesario for exemplary technical assistance, and Phil Jacobs for obtaining data on Alberta health expenditures. The authors maintain full responsibility for all interpretations or misinterpretations of policy activity.

CHAPTER 6

Reforming the British National Health Service: all change, no change?

WENDY RANADE

Introduction

The beginning of April 1991 was a defining moment for the British National Health Service when it embarked on a new trajectory of change. After a decade of ever more radical reforms of the public sector, the third Conservative administration headed by Mrs Thatcher introduced a sweeping set of changes into the NHS, the core of which was the establishment of an internal or quasi-market. Since then it has lived through six years of almost permanent upheaval. What has been achieved, and what are the prospects for the future, after a general election won by the Labour Party with a sweeping majority of 179 seats in Parliament in May 1997, after 18 years of opposition? This chapter explores the context and background to the health service reforms, their implementation and development, and assesses their impact six years on. It concludes by discussing how the new Labour Government propose to re-form the reforms, and the post-election prospects for the NHS.

The British health care system

The NHS is a publicly funded health system which is also, for the most part, publicly owned and operated. Funding is almost exclusively from taxation: 82 per cent direct taxes, 13 per cent payroll taxes and only 3 per cent direct charges (DOH, 1996a:13). Charges mainly cover prescribed drugs (at present £5.50 per item) but there are large exempt categories, and four-fifths of all prescriptions are dispensed free of charge to the consumer (Earl-Slater, 1996). Responsibility for hospitals and community health services in England rests with the Secretary of State for Health (and with the Welsh Secretary in Wales[1]), with authority to manage health services locally delegated to a system of appointed health authorities. Before 1991 these received cash-limited global budgets allocated according to a needs-based population formula to manage services in their area. Directly employed staff numbered 954,000 in 1991 (Government Statistical Service, 1996), but another 50,000 were contracted with the health service to supply general medical, dental, optical and pharmaceutical services. Of these, general practitioners (GPs), comprising 38 per cent of the medical workforce, deal with over 90 per cent of all patient contacts with the health service. Self-employed but publicly financed, they are funded on a capitation basis with extra payments for some specific services such as health promotion or antenatal clinics. Other primary health care staff were either directly employed by the GP or were attached to the practice as health authority employees (e.g. various kinds of community nursing staff). GPs have always safeguarded their independence, resisting being drawn into centralised health authority administration, and until April 1996 their contracts have always been administered by separate administrative bodies, the most recent of which were known as family health service authorities. Medical staff in hospitals, who are either salaried or work under contract, may work in both the public and private sectors.

The private acute medical sector is small but grew rapidly in the 1980s. In 1980, 6.4 per cent of the population had private medical insurance, which grew to 11.5 per cent by 1990 but this rose to 27 per cent of professionals and 23 per cent of employers and managers (Klein, 1995a: 155). Growth rates have been flat subsequently, in part due to the recession of the early 1990s, in part due to higher premiums and reducing waiting times in the NHS (*Financial Times*, 1997:1).

The British system has been described as 'meso-corporatist' (Moran, 1995), one where considerable powers of self-regulation and management were ceded by the state to the medical profession (over entry standards, discipline, clinical practice) and its influence over policy and resource allocation embedded within the NHS at every level through a variety of formal and informal mechanisms. In return doctors carried out the 'politically poisonous rationing decisions' (Harrison *et al.*, 1990:148) which a zero-priced system required. This happened at two levels: GPs acted as 'gatekeepers' to more expensive secondary and tertiary care; consultants allocated resources in hospitals, with the residual mismatch between demand and supply dealt with through waiting lists for treatment.

At a global level this concordat between the medical profession and the state worked well enough. Spending only 6 per cent of GNP on health care by 1988, Britain achieved health statistics comparable to countries spending much more, both as a percentage of GNP and per capita (see Table 1.1, ch. 1) but, as Moran (1995) notes, it was always an unstable system, since it tried to square a very difficult circle: universal access to 'comprehensive' medical care with limited funding. Its success also rested on certain conditions, notably a passive and deferential culture where patients accepted the 'objectivity' of medical decision making, and an expanding economy which could finance modest improvements in services over time.

Pressures for reform

The circumstances in which these arrangements began to break down are familiar and have been discussed at length elsewhere, notably by Klein (1995a) and Moran (1995). As in many other Western countries, growing demand pressures from an ageing population, rising citizen expectations and exploding medical technologies coincided with harsher economic conditions from the mid-1970s and a changing ideological climate to state welfare. The social and political deference which lubricated clinical rationing decisions in the past was fast disappearing as a result of growing affluence, exposure to health information in the media and higher educational standards. At the same time industrial relations within the NHS, traditionally peaceful and nonconflictual, worsened considerably between the years 1973 and 1982, with two national pay disputes and a number of others involving either specialised groups of staff (including medical staff) or disputes on local issues. Holding the lid on these demand pressures became increasingly problematic in the late 1970s given the parlous state of the British economy.

The formal break with Keynesian economic policies took place under Labour chancellors in 1975, who also introduced cash limits for health authority budgets to curb growth in spending, but the election of the first Conservative Government under Mrs Thatcher in 1979 signalled a tougher stance on public spending and an ideological break with the past. Under the influence of public choice economics, Mrs Thatcher had little respect for the 'bureau maximisers' and 'professional monopolists' of the welfare state, and was attracted to replacing a tax-funded NHS by a system of insurance (Timmins, 1996:392). In practice, however, Mrs Thatcher's radicalism was kept in check by Treasury opposition to any moves which would weaken its control over the public finances and its view that in international terms there was no better alternative to the NHS (Klein, 1995a:189). She also had to contend with the iconic status of the health service among the public. In opinion polls the NHS continues to be the most popular part of the welfare state, and majorities of 80 per cent or more consistently believe it merits higher levels of funding, even if this means paying higher taxes (Taylor-Gooby, 1995:4). The storm caused by a leaked Cabinet think-tank report in 1982, which floated the option of changing the funding system to one of private insurance, showed how great the political costs would be for any government which took such a measure, and within weeks of its publication Mrs. Thatcher felt bound to reassure the public at the Conservative Party Conference that '*The NHS is safe with us*'.

Professionalising management, managerialising the professions

Forced to maintain the fundamentals of the NHS, government attention turned instead to the way resources were used and the service managed. Apart from several low key measures to encourage the private medical sector and bring more private finance into the NHS, the main thrust of

Conservative policy in the 1980s was directed at improving the efficiency and management of the service. The techniques of the 'new public management' which the Conservatives were putting into place in the Civil Service were also applied to the NHS, in particular the delegation of financial management to lower levels; the emphasis on setting explicit targets of performance and holding managers accountable for results; new personnel management systems; and a relentless emphasis on the 'three E's' (economy, efficiency and effectiveness). Included in these measures was the imposition of staffing level targets and mandatory annual efficiency savings, to be partially achieved through programmes of compulsory competitive tendering in the ancillary services (catering, cleaning and laundries).

The most significant measure taken to professionalise management in these years was the appointment of general managers at all levels of the service, following the recommendations of the Griffith Report in 1983. Heading a small inquiry team of businessmen, Roy Griffiths (chief executive of the Sainsbury supermarket chain) argued that general managers, representing 'a more thrusting and committed style of management', should be given substantial discretionary freedom and a clearer policy steer from the centre (DHSS, 1983). To this end the central management of the service was reorganised, with a board chaired by the Secretary of State to provide policy direction and leadership, and a management board, headed by a Chief Executive of the NHS, responsible for implementation and the control of performance. (These are currently called the Policy Board and the NHS Executive.)

The Griffiths Report is significant for three reasons. It represented a break with the previous syndicalist and corporatist methods of management which allowed professional groups, notably doctors, the power to block change of which they disapproved. Secondly, it began the process by which doctors were to be made more aware of, and accountable for, the resource implications of their decisions, with workload-related budgets allocated to consultants on a pilot basis, in effect an attempt to managerialise the profession. Thirdly, it attacked the producer-led nature of the service, and argued for one which put the 'consumer' first.

The government's speedy implementation of the report's recommendations, barely four years after it had considered and rejected the general management model in another White Paper (DHSS, 1979), signifies a growing belief that the concordat between the medical profession and the state had outlived its utility, and was now under challenge through the attempt to empower a new set of 'corporate rationalisers' to do the government's bidding (Alford, 1975). General managers were not given the freedom from central prescription Griffiths had (perhaps naively) argued for and in practice their utility to government was as instruments to deliver increasingly tight financial targets (Harrison *et al.*, 1992; Strong and Robinson, 1990). Inevitably this brought managers into conflict with doctors, who showed little willingness to participate in resource management themselves and viewed the changes (rightly) as an attack on their professional autonomy. With few real powers of discipline and reward (for example, control over consultant contracts, pay or performance) most managers showed little inclination to engage doctors over issues of resource management or quality of care. Real increases in productivity and efficiency were achieved in the 1980s against a background of rigorous financial control (Robinson, 1991; Ranade and Haywood, 1991) but the heartlands of medical practice were left largely untouched, as demonstrated by the substantial variations that existed on every indicator of clinical practice.

By the 1987 election the financial pressures on the hospital and community health services were becoming politically unsustainable. Growth rates from 1980–81 to 1986–87 in this sector averaged less than one half per cent per year, at a time when growing demographic demands and the introduction of new technologies were estimated to require growth rates of 2 per cent per year in real terms (Appleby, 1992). The family health services, still demand-led and noncash-limited, had fared better, with real average increases of 3 per cent a year in the same period (Benzeval and Robinson, 1988). A financial crisis of unusual proportions precipitated a further review of the NHS, led by Mrs Thatcher in 1988. Once again radical options for changing the system of financing were considered and once again they were rejected. Attention turned instead to the organisational dynamics of the system and the way resources were allocated.

Reform proposals

The review group's proposals were outlined in a White Paper *Working for Patients* (WFP) (DOH, 1989a, 1989c) published in January 1989. This, together with a sister White Paper on community care, *Caring for People*, (DOH, 1989b) published a few months later, formed the basis of the NHS and Community Care Act of 1990. Many proposals consolidated and reinforced the managerialist trends of the previous decade, providing further tools for managers to discipline doctors and make medical practice more transparent and accountable. For instance, all doctors were required to participate in a system of medical audit which would be medically led but give managers some (weak) powers of oversight. Managers were also to be involved in the renegotiation of consultant contracts and merit awards[2] which for the first time required consultants to demonstrate 'not only their clinical skills but also a commitment to the management and development of the service' (DOH, 1989c:44). GPs were brought under more managerial control through the terms of a revised contract, imposed on an unwilling profession in 1990, as well as proposals in WFP. Together these established indicative prescribing budgets for GPs (not to be confused with the fundholding scheme, discussed below), required them to provide more services and information for patients, meet higher targets for vaccination and immunisation, and gave their administering bodies, family health service authorities, a more proactive and managerial role in planning and monitoring practice performance (for more details see Allsop, 1995: 207). Finally, smaller, more managerially oriented boards of directors were introduced for all health authorities and NHS trusts.

However the most contentious proposals were those which put in place an 'internal' or quasi-market (Le Grand and Bartlett, 1993) in which health authorities and GPs bought services on behalf of patients from NHS providers as well as the private and voluntary sector. An internal market for the NHS had first been suggested by the American economist Alain Enthoven, in a monograph he wrote after a study visit to the UK in 1984 (Enthoven, 1985). Like Griffiths before him, Enthoven argued that the NHS was producer-dominated and unresponsive to its users; change and innovation were difficult to effect and 'perverse incentives' positively penalised efficient management or clinical excellence, since there was no clear reward in extra resources. Various models of the quasi-market had subsequently been debated in academic and policy circles and the proposals outlined in WFP were an amalgam of different ideas. On the demand side, district health authorities (DHAs) were the primary purchasers of health services for their resident population and were given important responsibilities in assessing the health needs of them and seeing they were met. After a transition period they would receive budgets based on a weighted capitation formula and were free (within certain limits) to purchase services from a wider range of providers. GPs were the second category of purchasers. Eligible practices could opt to receive their practice budgets directly from the regional health authority to include a drug budget, 70 per cent of practice team staffing costs, improvements to premises and monies to buy a defined range of hospital treatments for their patients. (These were later extended to cover community health services as well.) Emergency and high cost services were specifically excluded. The cost of these services was deducted from the budget of the relevant DHA. Finally, the third category of purchaser was private patients and insurers.

Although all NHS providers were to be given greater autonomy to manage themselves, strongly managed hospitals and community health services could opt for self-governing status as NHS trusts, and were promised additional 'market' freedoms if they were successful, over staffing, pay, capital investment, and so on. They would compete for contracts from purchasers together with units still directly managed by health authorities, private and voluntary providers. In the theoretical model of the NHS quasi-market, competition would lever up standards of quality and efficiency; money would flow with the patient to reward the virtuous; the inefficient would go to the wall; and health authorities, since they were still cash-limited, would have a strong incentive to bargain hard to obtain greater value for money in health care on behalf of their residents. The only group which seemed to have little say in any of this were patients themselves, since although the reforms were paraded as providing 'greater consumer choice' they did nothing of the kind. Apart from finding it easier to change their GP, the public had no choice of their health agent, nor any way of influencing their decisions at a structural or strategic level. Far from 'money following the patient', as WFP proclaimed, patients would follow the contract with no more choice than before.

Predictions

Even within the confines of economic theory the outlook for the NHS market was not propitious, as Appleby makes clear in Chapter 3. The NHS was characterised by planned monopolies (to effect economies of scale), and was possibly the least pluralistic system in Western Europe. Information on costs, case mix, referral and patient flow patterns, quality of provision, outcomes and future needs was inadequate or rudimentary (Appleby *et al.*, 1994:37) and unlike in Sweden, little preparatory investment in improving requisite information systems was done in advance (Rehnberg, 1997). Poor information meant that at first DHAs had to set crude block contracts which simply specified access to a defined range of services in return for an annual fee, or block with 'ceilings and floors' which specified minimum and maximum levels of activity. According to economic theory, these would allow considerable scope for opportunism and 'games-playing' by providers which purchasers would find difficult to monitor (Light, 1990; Bartlett, 1991).

Le Grand and Bartlett (1993) suggested that as purchasers GPs better fitted the conditions specified for an efficient market than DHAs. They had better information on patient need, on the quality of care given by health care providers and the outcomes of treatment; satisfied the condition of contestability (even if in practice patients are reluctant to change their GPs); clearer financial incentives, and, as small businesspeople, a greater receptiveness to market signals. Balancing these considerations were the dangers of adverse selection, if GP fundholders removed high-cost patients from their lists or refused to take them on. Partial protection was provided by the fact that after £5,000 the DHA picked up the bill (later increased to £6,000) but the financial incentives remained. A detailed study of one GP practice showed that 5 per cent of patients accounted for 68 per cent of the total fundholding budget, and that such patients are easy to recognise from their medical histories (Glennerster *et al.*, 1994:104). The transaction costs of practice-based contracting were also likely to be much higher than DHA purchasing.

Implementation and policy development

The reforms were implemented in a climate of both public and professional hostility within very tight timescales, allowing only 18 months before the date on which the new contracting arrangements went 'live'. Within months it became apparent that the neoclassical concept of the market, implicit in WFP, was unworkable in the NHS. Providing a stable environment for the new trusts was seen as the overriding priority, which led to a slowdown in the pace of change, heavier regulation and a partial return to planning. Ministers also intervened to protect London's health services, when market pressures threatened to close some of the capital's hospitals, and instituted a major planning enquiry on their future (Tomlinson, 1992). The results of this are now being implemented, with major rationalisations of acute services and substantial investment in primary and community care.

In other ways too, market freedoms were heavily curbed. To prevent monopoly abuse, trusts were already limited to a 6 per cent return on assets, and prices must be set to equal short-run average cost for each speciality. No cross-subsidisation between different buyers or products is meant to occur (difficult to enforce in practice however). Income and expenditure must balance, 'taking one year with another', and there is no automatic right to carry forward surpluses or make deficits. Their promised freedom to borrow capital, which had been an important motivating factor in applications for trust status, was also severely constrained in practice by setting tight external financing limits (EFLs) – in effect a cash limit on total capital and revenue expenditure – in the interests of Treasury expenditure control. Although no longer bound by centrally negotiated pay agreements for staff, moving towards a system of local pay proved complex and contentious, and has not been fully achieved.

Early case study evidence in the West Midlands Region suggested that progressive managers in the NHS hoped to develop a 'relational' market based on longer term partnerships with preferred providers, and competition replaced by contestability (see Chapter 3; see also Ranade, 1994; Robinson and Le Grand, 1995; Ferlie *et al.*, 1996). Such a model was perceived to be more appropriate to the complexities and uncertainties of health care, and reduced transaction costs. Evidence that the DOH had caught up with this thinking came in a succession of speeches on purchasing in 1993 by the Health Minister where the previous emphasis on purchasers promoting provider competition was replaced by an emphasis on the maintenance of 'mature relations', 'partnerships and long-term agreements' with providers (Mawhinney, 1993).

Two other aspects of implementation also merit attention. First, the unexpected growth in NHS Trusts and GP fundholders, both of which were largely experimental aspects of the reforms. Fifty-seven units accounting for 13.5 per cent of total NHS expenditure began operating as trusts in the first wave from April 1991; by April 1994 trusts accounted for 95 per cent of expenditure and have now become the accepted management model for the NHS. Similarly, the first phase of fundholding accounted for 300 practices and 7.5 per cent of the population but this steadily increased to cover over half the population by 1996 (Audit Commission, 1996). Applicants were at first restricted to larger practices with list sizes in excess of 9,000 patients, later reduced to 7,000. Since then further work has facilitated the entry of even smaller practices by grouping them into consortia or multifunds. One-third of practices entering the scheme were grouped in this way in 1995–96 compared to only 2 per cent of first wave practices in 1991–92 (Audit Commission, 1996:17).

A second notable feature of the reforms was the extent to which implementation was 'bottom-up' and shaped by the implementors themselves. The NHS has always been characterised by pendulum swings between bouts of centralisation (to satisfy public accountability requirements) and a decentralising reaction against the rigidities this causes (Klein, 1995a; Ham, 1992a:169–74). Although centralising tendences dominated the 1980s, in introducing a quasi-market into the NHS, ministers and the DOH were entering unknown territory as they openly admitted and managers had to be given discretion to shape the reforms to fit local circumstances. The most visible aspect of this was the creation of consortia arrangements between purchasers and alliances between DHAs and FHSAs, the administrative bodies for primary care. Legislation followed to formalise these alliances, and in April 1996 new integrated health authorities, combining the functions of the two previous authorities, started work. Meanwhile a wave of trust mergers and realignments also took place.

This frenzy of interorganisational restructuring was paralleled by experiments in decentralised commissioning of services, either based on geographical localities or groups of GP practices. The motives were various: to involve GPs in purchasing decisions in a bid to woo them away from fundholding; to draw together fundholders and nonfundholders in more cooperative partnerships in an attempt to prevent inequities between the two groups developing; to become more informed about local needs; to involve local communities in the development of service specifications, placing and monitoring of contracts (Balogh, 1996; Ham, 1992b; Higgins and Girling, 1994). Occasionally there was a more radical agenda. Health authorities had been exhorted by the NHS Executive to become 'champions of the people' and consult closely with local people in commissioning of services and setting contracts (DOH, 1990; NHS Management Executive, 1992). Some authorities used this to empower local users and strengthen mechanisms of citizen participation. This may take the form of supporting vulnerable groups such as mental health services users to have an input into service planning and monitoring. In other cases health authorities and trusts have worked in partnership with other agencies such as local authorities, voluntary and self-help groups on initiatives around urban regeneration and health, which are explicitly modelled on community development principles of empowerment (e.g. Sandwell Health Authority in the West Midlands). The initiatives were interesting in showing how the mechanisms created by the reforms could be used in the service of an alternative agenda and set of values.

From 1994 the DOH announced that primary care would in future take the lead in purchasing, as well as a major expansion of the fundholding scheme. This included trials in total fundholding, where individual or groups of practices could opt to hold the budget for all the services they required, including emergency care. As Balogh (1996) points out, one effect has been that more recent experiments in locality purchasing and commissioning have concentrated primarily on GPs to the exclusion of other stakeholders, in acknowledgement of the thrust of policy and the shifting balance of power which is putting GPs in the driving seat of change.

Assessment

The difficulties of assessing reform outcomes six years later are considerable (see Pollitt, 1995 for an extended discussion of the methodological problems involved). The reforms have been subject to almost continuous policy development which has introduced numerous confounding factors, including the effects of parsimonious or generous budget settlements in different years, organisational restructuring and the impact of new responsibilities and tasks, notably after the Patient's Charter and the *Health of the Nation* White Paper were published in 1992 (DOH, 1991, 1992). The former set out 27 national health targets in five key areas such as coronary health disease and cancers; the latter set out standards which patients had a right to expect on service aspects, like waiting times, which were continuously reviewed and improved. Considerable political energy has been put into the achievement of these targets and they are written into the performance contracts of health authorities.

Other developments were driven by wider technological, economic or demographic forces and would have happened anyway, although perhaps not at such a fast pace, such as the move towards a 'primary care-led service' (NHSE, 1994). In addition, several elements of the reforms have been poorly researched, and the government itself has not undertaken any systematic evaluation. Fundholding has probably attracted most research attention (reviewed in Dixon and Glennerster, 1995), including a recent major study by the Audit Commission (1996). Given these caveats, the next section assesses the available evidence.

Outcomes

Efficiency and effectiveness

Evidence of improvements in productive efficiency is ambiguous. The government points to activity data, citing an increase of 18 per cent in 'finished consultant episodes' between 1990–91 and 1993–94 (with a further 6.5 per cent increase the following year) and a doubling of day cases between 1990–91 and 1994–95, achieved against a backdrop of reducing numbers of available beds (from 7.1 per 1,000 population in 1984 to 4.3 per thousand in 1994–95) (DOH, 1996a; BMJ, 1996). These increases coincided with two years of unusually generous budget settlements, however (6.1 per cent in real terms in 1991–92, and 5.5 per cent in 1992–93) and rapid technological improvements which allowed a greater proportion of surgical work to be carried out on a day surgery basis.

Newchurch and Company Health Service Briefing (1995) argue that in crude activity terms nursing productivity rose by 20 per cent whilst the nursing workforce fell by 4 per cent between 1988 and 1992, although these figures may also be distorted by changes in service configuration and contracting out. In cost terms nursing productivity stood still, reflecting substantial increases in nursing pay over this period (*Ibid.*). The productivity of medical staff increased by only 2 per cent in activity terms over the same period, but in cost terms actually declined, reflecting a 12.5 per cent increase in staff over the same period (Newchurch and Company Health Service Briefing, 1995:3).

Efficiency savings made by GP fundholders were estimated at £206 million up to March 1995 by the Audit Commission, largely derived from more cost-effective prescribing of drugs, more appropriate referral practices, reductions in inappropriate outpatient attendances and making budget savings (Audit Commission 1996:60–61; see also Penhale *et al.*, 1993; Coulter and Bradlow, 1993). Efficiency savings were, however, outweighed by the £232 million received by fundholders in the same period to cover the costs of management, information technology and administration. In addition the direct costs of administering the scheme by FHSAs were estimated to average £6,600 per fund (Audit Commission, 1996: 66).

An important strand of policy development has been the increased emphasis on clinical effectiveness and cost effectiveness, which partly derives, as Robinson points out, from the enhanced role of public health medicine in assessing health needs and in the purchasing function (Robinson, 1996:338). A national research and development strategy for the NHS to improve information to support this development began in 1991, with the establishment of a number of national and regional bodies to coordinate work on clinical guidelines and to commission, review and disseminate research. Purchasers have been given the responsibility for implementing 'evidence-based medicine' through their contracts (NHS Management Executive, 1996) but analysing, assessing and prioritising the results of research in relation to local needs continues to be a daunting task.

Contracting

By 1994–95 block contracts were still the predominant national model but 69 per cent incorporated more sophisticated risk management procedures, displaying some of the characteristics of relational contracts (Robinson, 1996). Pricing structures still seem to be cost-led and a recent analysis of all the contracts set by eight health authorities found tenfold variations in prices which currently prevail for the same items of service (Roberts *et al.*, 1996). This finding lends weight to the need to develop more open and standardised pricing procedures as a matter of urgency (Robinson and Le Grand, 1995).

Transaction costs have proved to be considerable, as predicted, with many complaints about the time-consuming nature of the annual contract negotiations between health authorities and trusts, but little good evidence on the direct or indirect costs. The transaction costs of dealing with services which fall outside the main contracts and are dealt with as extracontractual referrals seem particularly high (Ghodse, 1995; Maheswaran *et al.*, 1994) as do those associated with GP purchasing. GPs use more cost per case contracts and trusts have to deal with multiple purchasers. The cost of dealing with each fundholding practice was estimated at £12,500 for each community trust, £8,000 for each acute trust in 1996 by the NHS Trust Federation (*Health Service Journal*, 1996).

Labour Party critics of the quasi-market pointed to the rapid expansion in the number of managers in the NHS (up by 10,000 between 1990 and 1993) as further evidence of high transaction costs. However, the rise is difficult to interpret (Appleby, 1995) and managers still account for only 3 per cent of directly employed staff.

Competition

In spite of studies which purport to show the potential competitiveness of several important acute specialities (Appleby *et al.*, 1994), actual competition depends on the behaviour of purchasers and providers and seems in practice to be quite limited. The inability of trusts to carry forward surpluses and build reserves, and the imposition of annual efficiency savings across the board on all trusts, decreases the incentives for long-term productive efficiency gains, reduces the gain to any hospital of cutting margins, and therefore weakens the incentives for providers to respond to competitive pressures (Propper, 1995). On the purchasing side, GP fundholders appear to have been more successful than DHA purchasers in stimulating competition by seeking out alternative providers and have shown greater willingness to experiment with service patterns, for example, developing consultant outreach clinics, and providing a wider range of community services on the practice premises such as physiotherapy, dietetics and counselling (Audit Commission, 1996; Glennerster *et al.*, 1994; National Audit Office, 1994).

Impact on patients

Waiting times have been reduced over the past five years, with significant cuts in the longest waiting times. Two year waits were eliminated by the first set of Patient's Charter targets, and those waiting a year or more for inpatient treatment have been reduced from 200,000 to less than 5,000 (2 per cent of the waiting list total) by March 1996. Recently, however, waiting list totals have climbed again to an all-time high of 1.1 million, with a small increase in those waiting over one year. This probably reflects the tough financial settlement the NHS received in 1996–97 (0.9 per cent in real terms) and a 4 per cent winter rise in emergency admissions (Timmins, 1997).

Direct research evidence of the reforms' impact on patients is summarised in Robinson and Le Grand (1994) but this only covers the early years (up to 1993). On consumer choice there was little evidence that patients had any greater choice of hospital or consultant (Mahon *et al.*, 1994; Jones *et al.*, 1994) and they are reluctant to exercise their choice to change GPs.

On quality and responsiveness the evidence is mixed and often anecdotal. It is probably fair to say that where quality improvements have been linked to special funding, Patient's Charter performance targets or other high profile central initiatives, such as the implementation of the Cumberledge Report on maternity services (DOH, 1993), improvements have been achieved by DHA purchasers. Early research on fundholders suggested they were more successful in improving the choice and quality of services available for their patients (Glennerster *et al.*, 1994; National Audit Office, 1994). The Audit Commission (1996) confirmed that a substantial majority of fundholders had achieved reduced waiting times in most specialities, improved local access to certain services, and better standards of nonclinical care for their patients. Significantly only a minority offered patients a choice of provider depending on the individual's wishes.

Equity concerns have focused chiefly on GP fundholders, who were perceived as having been treated generously at the expense of nonfundholders, allowing them to negotiate shorter waiting times, or better services for their patients. This replaced earlier concerns that fundholders would underserve their patients, which did not appear to materialise (*Health Service Journal*, 1995; Audit Commission, 1996; Whitehead, 1994). Similarly there is no evidence that 'cream skimming' has occurred on a systematic basis, although individual incidents have appeared in the press (Audit Commission 1996: 106). Moves towards a uniform system of weighted capitation budgets for fundholders (adjusted for age and sex of patients on the practice list) are only now being implemented.

Are patients more satisfied with the services they receive? Once again interpreting the evidence is not easy. In opinion polls, those dissatisfied with the NHS fell from a peak of 46 per cent in 1989 to 38 per cent in 1994 (Moore, 1996), but such surveys tell us more about the current state of media coverage of the NHS than they do about the quality of services. Patients themselves often record very high levels of satisfaction with overall levels of care which is belied by responses on particular issues (Moore, 1996). Complaints to community health councils (the body which represents patient's interests in each district) have doubled between 1990 and 1994, as have those to the Health Service Ombudsman. This could either mean quality is declining or people are less inclined to accept poor standards, and are encouraged not to by the Patient's Charter.

System effects

At a systems level, the reforms have profoundly unsettled the previous equilibrium and the way the system functions, creating new paradoxes and points of tension. The first centres on the tension between centralism and devolution, to which I have already referred. Although managers have gained considerable autonomy at the operational level, this is combined with a centralisation of policy through the NHS Executive, which increasingly sets the strategic objectives for the NHS and delineates the methods of achieving them. Annual performance contracts with health authorities are enforced through a simplified line of hierarchical control to the centre (with the abolition of regional health authorities and their replacement by eight regional offices of the NHS Executive in 1996) and these objectives and targets are in turn imposed on providers through the mechanism of purchasing contracts. At the same time the lessening of *direct* controls over trusts has been accompanied by an extension of 'arms length' forms of monitoring and evaluation through the increasing use of published performance league tables (e.g. on waiting times), and the extension of methods of audit and evaluation through bodies like the Audit Commission. Increasingly, therefore, the outcome of the reforms seems less like a 'market' and more like a new system of performance management.

Greater operational autonomy, combined with different performance incentives, have released a great deal of managerial and clinical creativity and innovation. In this sense the reforms have had a cathartic effect on the NHS, breaking down service barriers and rigid personnel practices which previously seemed impossible to change. But the downside of this diversity and experiment is complexity and fragmentation. The system has become more difficult to understand or to steer in a coherent strategic direction, and this is the second source of tension and role conflict. For example, in the new 'primary care-led' NHS, health authorities are slowly relinquishing responsibility for direct purchasing to GPs but continue to be responsible for developing and implementing local health strategies to improve the health of their local population (NHS Management Executive, 1994). This requires the agreement and cooperation of GPs, trusts, and other stakeholders over whom the the authority has either limited or no direct control (e.g. local authorities or the private sector). Managers, therefore, have to learn to achieve change through increasingly complex networks, as well as through markets and hierachies.

Finally, old power struggles between doctors and managers have been overlaid by the new organisational schism of purchasers and providers in the quasi-market, and complex shifts in the power of different groups, the outcome of which is still far from resolved. Competitive incentives and sanctions seemed to lead to more corporate working between managers and doctors in NHS trusts at first (Ranade, 1995), if only to ensure corporate survival, with the internal organisation and management of hospitals increasingly based on clinical directorates for a speciality or group of specialities. Clinical directors aided by business managers have delegated budgets and are responsible for workloads, contract negotiations, quality of care issues, and so on. However, the cooption of doctors into management has not taken place willingly and it is far from clear how it will evolve.

The most significant shift in power has clearly been from doctors in hospitals to doctors in primary care, yet this too has had contradictory effects. GPs have been given greater decision-making power over the planning and commissioning of services and control of budgets, but the price has been losing some of their cherished administrative independence. Bringing them into the NHS mainstream, and making them more accountable to health authorities, has made them more susceptible to managerial control. The surveillance of the effectiveness of hospital clinical practice by GPs (and public health physicians in health authorities) is gradually demystifying hospital medicine, and making it more transparent and accountable, but GPs are also caught up in the same web of pressures to practise 'evidence-based medicine' themselves. If fundholding develops into fully fledged 'managed care' organisations, led by GPs and delivering or commissioning a comprehensive set of primary, secondary and community health services for their patients (Maynard, 1996) they would be accountable to, and under contract with, health authorities. The sanctions and incentives for GPs to practise in a cost-effective manner would be reinforced, and make them the chief rationers of care.

A new government, a converging agenda

A new Labour government was returned to office in May 1997, with a majority much larger than expected. Before the election the Party's proposals for the NHS were relatively modest and set out most fully in *Renewing the NHS* (Labour Party, 1995), amplified by an important speech by the Shadow Secretary of State in November 1996 (Smith, 1996). Labour's stance reflected its own repositioning under its new leader, Tony Blair, as a centre-left social democratic party, which has jettisoned much ideological baggage from the past. This applies to the health reforms as well, and most of the substance, it seemed, would remain. Although the Labour Party was pledged to get rid of the 'internal market', the only clear proposal to do so was the abolition of GP fundholding. Underneath the rhetoric and renaming taking place, the main planks of the reforms – the purchaser–provider split, contracts, NHS trusts, the emphasis on primary care and 'evidence-based medicine' – stayed.

The Party proposed replacing individual practice-based GP fundholding by local commissioning groups led by GPs, based on existing decentralised models already referred to earlier in the chapter. Five to 15 groups were envisaged for each authority, who would commission most of the services they needed from their delegated share of the health authority budget. Health authorities (fewer and larger) would concentrate on strategic planning, public health, supporting and developing GP commissioning and primary care, resource allocation and performance monitoring. Any quality improvements would have to be found from efficiency savings. There were many hopes of reducing transaction costs by the abolition of fundholding, moving to longer term contracts, and other measures to simplify the contracting process in order to take a further 100,000 patients off the waiting lists. How far these proposals will reduce 'bureaucracy' and release resources is open to challenge, but with the Labour Chancellor taking an even stricter line than the Conservatives on taxation and public spending, it is clear that resource pressures in the NHS will continue to be intense.

What is unclear since the election is how far the new government will feel they now have a mandate for more radical change. The new Secretary of State, Frank Dobson, has stopped the eighth wave of fundholding, but is seeking fuller consultation on other proposals and once more reviewing financing options. Meanwhile, some observers are urging the abolition of the purchaser–provider split (Paton, 1997) and there is a wider scepticism that the proposal on local commissioning groups would save on administration and transaction costs.

In other ways there are clear signs that the party wants to use the mechanisms of the reforms to promote a different agenda and set of values to restore a more equitable and less fragmented service. Public health concerns would be tackled more vigorously by the newly created Minister for Public Health (a White Paper on banning tobacco advertising and sports sponsorship, and promoting other antismoking measures is promised soon) and the party plans to have a new enquiry into health inequalities to update the seminal Black Report of 1980 (*Health Service Journal*, 1997).

Conclusions

When the Conservatives embarked on the NHS reforms in 1989 they unleashed an ideological crusade on the NHS which seemed like a deliberate exercise in destabilisation for its own sake, with no clear goals in sight. Then Health Minister David Mellor, for example, declared at the time he had 'no idea what the NHS would look like in five or six years time' (Butler, 1992:48). Since then it has lived through its own permanent revolution: 'an institution which is constantly reinventing itself [like] a car that is being re-engineered even while it is roaring round on the test track' (Klein, 1995b:101). The government were widely criticised in 1989 for launching untried proposals on the NHS nationally without pilots or evaluation but, ironically, the reforms have given rise to an unprecedented degree of policy learning and innovation, with pilots and experiments of all kinds flourishing. (Trust status and GP fundholding were, after all, voluntary even if in practice this was accompanied by strong central 'persuasion' and generous financial inducements.)

Revolution is now giving way to evolution, and a more pragmatic and careful exploration of ways forward. Nothing better illustrates this change than a recent Conservative White Paper (DOH, 1996b) which pushes the primary care revolution further by proposing changes in the GP contract to enable more flexible ways of organising and providing services. In utter contrast to *Working for Patients* (DOH, 1989), this White Paper was based on months of consultation, and all its proposals are for piloting and evaluation first. Even before the election it was possible to discern a new consensus on the way forward, based on a retreat from competition and markets in favour of a 'primary care-led service' and 'evidence-based medicine' as the new panaceas. But restructuring health services and persuading clinicians to change their behaviour even when the evidence is (unusually) clear-cut, is proving to be a daunting, and uphill task: there are no quick fixes, and the benefits may not be forthcoming quickly enough to satisfy politicians facing short-term financial or media pressures.

The big question for the future therefore still relates to funding. Can a 'comprehensive' health service continue to be provided on the basis of tax-funding when both parties are staking their credibility so clearly on a low tax regime? Both Labour and Conservatives have pledged themselves to a comprehensive service (politically they could do no other before an election) and argue that the rationing dilemma is no greater today than it has ever been in the history of the NHS (see, for instance, DOH, 1996c; Smith, 1996).

Yet the definition of 'comprehensive' is already being narrowed. Optical services and large sections of dentistry have been privatised with no promise of restoration by the Labour Party. Responsibility for long-stay nursing care has been transferred from the NHS, where it was free, to local authorities, where it is means tested and largely provided by the private sector. The Conservative election manifesto contained proposals to push long-stay and social care futher down the privatisation road, with schemes for private insurance and the transfer of all provision to the independent sector. Local authorities would still have a lead role but only in assessing needs and purchasing services to meet them, not as providers.

Some commentators argue this could be a model for the health service too in future, if financial pressures were perceived to be unsupportable (see, for instance, Hunter, 1997). At present such a suggestion seems fanciful and is not on the current or future agenda of the Labour Party, although there are many on the radical right of the Conservative Party who would see this as the logical consequence of the Thatcherite revolution. Ironically the translation of the 'patient' into the 'consumer' in the internal market, with explicit rights set out in the Patient's Charter, has fuelled user expectations about the quality of public services, and much will be expected from a Labour Government, yet it has promised to do no more than fund the NHS to keep pace with inflation. We can, therefore, fairly confidently predict that funding 'crises' will figure as often on the agenda of the next government as they have in previous ones. In that sense it is 'all change, no change' in the new model NHS.

Notes

1. Responsibility for the NHS in Scotland and Northern Ireland is vested in the respective Secretaries of State for Scotland and Northern Ireland. In general the policies outlined in the chapter apply to the four countries of the United Kingdom although Scotland has always had separate legislation, and Northern Ireland has rather different administrative arrangements to the other three.

2. Merit or distinction awards are a permanent addition to a consultant's salary, awarded for 'distinguished' service.

References

Alford, R. R. (1975) *Health Care Politics: Ideological and Interest Group Barriers to Reform*, Chicago: University of Chicago Press.

Allsop, J. (1995) *Health Policy and the NHS: Towards 2000*, 2nd edn, London: Longman.

Appleby, J. (1992) *Financing Health Care in the 1990s*, Buckingham: Open University Press.

Appleby, J. (1995) 'Managers in the ascendancy', *Health Service Journal*, 21 September, **105** (5471):32–33.

Appleby, J., Little, V., Ranade, W., Robinsons, R. and Smith, P. (1994) 'Monitoring managed competition' in R. Robinson and J. Le Grand (eds) *Evaluating the NHS Reforms*, London: King's Fund Institute.

Audit Commission (1996) *What the Doctor Ordered: A Study of GP Fundholders in England and Wales*, London: HMSO.

Balogh, R. (1996) 'Exploring the role of localities in health commissioning: A review of the literature', *Social Policy and Administration*, **30**(2): 99–113.

Bartlett, W. (1991) 'Quasi-markets and contracts: A markets and hierarchies perspective on NHS reforms', *Public Money and Management*, **1**(3):53–60.

Benzeval, M. and Robinson, R. (1988) *Health Care Finance: Assessing the Options*, Briefing Paper 4, London: King's Fund Institute.

Black, Sir D. (1980) *Inequalities in Health: Report of a Research Working Group*, London: DHSS.

British Medical Journal (1996) '20 per cent increase in four years', **313**:103.

Butler, J. (1992) *Patients, Policies and Politics: Before and After Working for Patients*, Buckingham: Open University Press.

Coulter. A. and Bradlow, J. (1993) 'Effects of NHS reforms on general practitioners' referral patterns', *British Medical Journal*, **306**:433–7.

Department of Health (1989a) *Working for Patients*, Cm 555, London: HMSO.

Department of Health (1989b) *Caring for People*, Cm 7615, London: HMSO.

Department of Health (1989c) *Working for Patients: Medical Audit Working Paper, 6*, London: HMSO.

Department of Health (1990) *Developing Districts*, London: HMSO.

Department of Health (1991) *The Patient's Charter*, London: HMSO.

Department of Health (1992) *The Health of the Nation*, Cm 1986, London: HMSO.

Department of Health (1993) *Changing Childbirth: Report of the Expert Maternity Group* (Cumberledge Report), London: HMSO.

Department of Health (1996a) *Health and Personal Social Service Statistics for England* 1995, London: HMSO.

Department of Health (1996b) *Primary Care the Future: Choice and Opportunity*, London: HMSO.

Department of Health (1996c) *A Service with Ambitions*, London: HMSO.

Department of Health and Social Security (1979) *Patients First*, London: HMSO.

Department of Health and Social Security (1983) *Inquiry into NHS Management* (The Griffiths Report), London:HMSO.

Developing NHS Purchasing and GP fundholding (EL(94)79) October.

Dixon, J. and Glennerster, H. (1995) 'What do we know about fundholding in general practice?', *British Medical Journal*, **311**: 727–30.

Earl-Slater, A. (1996) 'Privatising medicine in the National Health Service', *Public Money and Management*, **16**(2): 39–44.

Enthoven, A. (1985) *Reflections on the Management of the National Health Service*, London: Nuffield Provincial Hospitals Trust.

Ferlie, E, Pettigrew, A., Ashburner, L. and Fitzgerald, L. (1996) *The New Public Management in Action*, Oxford: Oxford University Press.

Financial Times (1997) 'Private medical insurance: *Financial Times* Survey', 23 May, pp. 1–4.

Ghodse, B. (1995) 'Extra-contractual referrals: safety valve or administrative paper chase', *British Medical Journal*, **310**: 1573–6.

Glennerster, H., Matsaganis, M. and Owens, P. (1994) *Implementing GP Fundholding: Wild Card or Winning Hand?*, Buckingham: Open University Press.

Government Statistical Service (1996) *Social Trends 26*, London: HMSO.

Ham, C. (1992a) *Health Policy in Britain*, 3rd edn, Basingstoke: Macmillan

Ham, C. (1992b) *Locality Purchasing*, Discussion Paper 30, Health Services Management Centre, University of Birmingham.

Harrison, S., Hunter, D. and Pollitt, C. (1990) *The Dynamics of British Health Policy*, London: Unwin Hyman.

Harrison, S., Hunter, D., Marnoch, G. and Pollitt, C. (1992*) Just Managing: Power and Culture in the National Health Service*, London: Macmillan.

Health Service Journal (1995) 'Fundholders are not putting cash before care', **105** (5444):6.

Health Service Journal (1996) 'Jobs will go in drive to cut red tape', **106** (5504):3.

Health Service Journal (1997) 'Labour government would set up inquiry into health inequalities', **107** (5546):7.

Higgins, J. and Girling, J. (1994) 'Purchasing for health: the development of an idea', in A. Harrison (ed.) *Health Care U.K. 1994–94*, London: King's Fund Institute.

Hunter, D. (1997) 'Prepare for a future shock', *Health Service Journal*, **107** (5546):24.

Jones, D., Lester, C. and West, R. (1994) 'Monitoring changes in health services for older people', in R. Robinson and J. Le Grand (eds) *Evaluating the NHS Reforms*, London: King's Fund Institute.

Klein, R. (1995a) *The New Politics of the NHS*, 3rd edn, London: Longman.

Klein, R. (1995b) 'Learning from others', Paper given to Four Country Conference in Health Care Reforms and Health Care Policies in the United States, Canada, Germany and the Netherlands. Rotterdam, February.

Labour Party (1995) *Renewing the NHS*, London: Labour Party Central Office.

Le Grand, J. and Bartlett, W. (1993) *Quasi-markets and Social Policy*, London: Macmillan.

Light, D. (1990) 'Learning from their mistakes', *Health Service Journal*, **99** (5148):1–2.

Maheswaran, S., Weil, J. and Munday, S. (1994) 'Heavyweight', *Health Service Journal*, **104**: 32.

Mahon, A., Wilkin, D. and Whitehouse, C. (1994) 'Choice of hospital for elective surgery referral: GPs and patients' views' in R. Robinson and J. Le Grand (eds) *Evaluating the NHS Reforms*, London: King's Fund Institute.

Mawhinney, B. (1993) *Purchasing for Health: A Framework for Action*, Leeds: NHS Management Executive.

Maynard, A. (1996) 'At the leading edge', *Health Service Journal*, **106** (5500):25.

Moore, W. (1996) 'And how are we feeling today?', *Health Service Journal*, **106** (5495): 30–32.

Moran, M. (1995) 'Explaining change in the National Health Service: Corporatism, closure and democratic capitalism', *Public Policy and Administration*, **10** (2):21–34.

National Audit Office (1994) *General Practitioner Fundholding in England*, London: HMSO.

Newchurch and Company Health Service Briefing (1995) *Strategic Change in the NHS 3 – Acute Services: A Prognosis for the Millenium*, London: Newchurch.

NHS Management Executive (1992) *Local Voices: The Views of Local People in Purchasing for Health*, EL (1992) 1.

NHS Management Executive (1994) *Developing NHS Purchasing and GP Fundholding: Towards a Primary Care-led NHS*.

NHS Management Executive (1996) *Priorities and Planning Guidance for 1995–96*, EL(94)55.

Paton, C. (1997) 'The future in your hands', *Health Service Journal*, 8 May, p.18.

Penhale, D. *et al.* (1993) 'A comparison of first-wave fundholding and non-fundholding practices', Unpublished manuscript, City University.

Pollit, C. (1995) 'Justification by works or by faith? Evaluating the new public management', *Evaluation*, **1**(2):133–54.

Pritchard, C. (1992) 'What can we afford for the National Health Service?', *Social Policy and Administration*, **26**(1):40–54.

Propper, C. (1995) 'Regulatory reform of the NHS internal market', *Health Economics*, **4**: 77–83.

Raferty, J., Robinson, R., Malgan, J. and Forrest, S. (1996) 'Contracting in the NHS quasi-market', *Health Economics*, 1996.

Ranade, W (1994) *A Future for the NHS? Health Care in the 1990s*, London: Longman.

Ranade, W. (1995) 'The theory and practice of managed competition in the NHS, *Public Administration*, **73** (2):243–63.

Ranade, W. and Haywood, S. (1991) 'Privatising from within: The National Health Service under Thatcher', in C. Altenstetter and S. Haywood (eds) *From Rhetoric to Reality: Healthcare and the New Right*, London: Macmillan.

Rehnberg, C. (1997) 'Sweden', in C. Ham (ed.) *Health Care Reform*, Buckingham: Open University Press.

Roberts, C. *et al.*, (1996) 'The wasted millions', *Health Service Journal*, **106** (5525):24–27.

Robinson, R. (1991) 'Health expenditures: Recent trends and prospects for the 1990s', *Public Money and Management*, **11**(4):19–24.

Robinson, R. (1996) 'The impact of the NHS reforms 1991–1995: a review of research evidence', *Journal of Public Health Medicine*, **18**(3):337–42.

Robinson, R., and Le Grand, J. (1994) *Evaluating the NHS Reforms*, London: King's Fund Institute.

Robinson, R. and Le Grand, J. (1995) 'Contracting and the purchaser–provider split', in R. Saltman and C. von Otter (eds) *Implementing Planned Markets in Health Care*, Buckingham: Open University Press.

Smith, C. (1996) 'A Health Service for a New Century: Labour's proposals to replace the internal market in the NHS', Speech by Shadow Secretary of Health, 3rd December.

Strong, P. M. and Robinson, J. (1990) *The NHS – Under New Management*, Buckingham: Open University Press.

Taylor-Gooby, P (1995) 'Comfortable, marginal and excluded: Who should pay higher taxes for a better welfare state?' in R. Jowell, J. Curtice, A. Park, L. Brook and D. Ahrendt (eds) *British Social Attitudes, The 12th Report*, Aldershot: Dartmouth.

Timmins, N. (1996*) The Five Giants: A Biography of the Welfare State*, London: Fontana.

Timmins, N. (1997) 'Hospital waiting lists reach 1.1 million record in England', *Financial Times*, 20 February, p. 1.

Tomlinson, Sir B. (1992) *Report of the Inquiry into London's Health Services, Medical Education and Research*, London: Department of Health.

Whitehead, M. (1994) 'Is it fair? Evaluating the equity implications of the reforms', in R. Robinson and J. Le Grand (eds) *Evaluating the NHS Reforms*, London: King's Fund Institute.

CHAPTER 7

Reforming New Zealand health care

JACQUELINE CUMMING and
GEORGE SALMOND

Introduction

In July 1991, the New Zealand government announced a package of health reform proposals designed to transform New Zealand's health care system. These proposals were based around a framework of managed competition, with competition in both purchasing and provision to promote efficiency and responsiveness.

In this chapter, we analyse key developments in New Zealand health policy since 1991. We begin by briefly discussing pressures for reform. The 1991 reform proposals and their implementation are then described. The chapter discusses how the reforms have worked in practice and provides an overview of reform outcomes, with a particular emphasis on primary care and secondary care medical and surgical services. We conclude with a discussion on New Zealand's overall experience with the health reforms and the sector's likely future directions.

Pressures for reform

Two broad sets of pressures have contributed to both the desire and the form of health care reform in New Zealand in the 1990s.

Internal pressures: the structure of New Zealand health care to 1980

By the early 1980s, New Zealand's health care system consisted of four[1] sets of institutional arrangements for the funding and delivery of health care. (See Table 7.1 for statistical data relating to this discussion.)

In primary care, the traditional form of payment has been fee-for-service government subsidies to independent general practitioners (GPs), specialists and other professionals, and for pharmaceuticals. Historically, all New Zealanders have been eligible for such subsidies. GPs act as gatekeepers for access to subsidised pharmaceutical and laboratory services, as well as to secondary (hospital) services.

New Zealanders have had free access to hospital care since 1938. Publicly owned hospitals – governed by locally elected boards but

Table 7.1 *The New Zealand health sector: a statistical overview*

	1980	1984	1988	1991	1992	1993	1994	1995	Change 1980–84	1984–88	1988–92	1991–93	1993–95
Expenditure													
Total nominal expenditure ($ million)	1,382	2,244	4,299	5,394	5,662	5,843	6,086	6,444	62.37%	91.58%	31.71%	8.32%	10.29%
Total real expenditure per capita ($1,995)(CPI adjusted)	1,488	1,439	1,655	1,707	1,750	1,766	1,795	1,814	-3.29%	15.01%	5.74%	3.46%	2.72%
Public funding as a % of total funding	88	87	85.62	82.24	79.03	76.58	76.8	76.87	-1.14%	-1.59%	-7.70%	-6.88%	0.38%
Private household expenditure as a % of total expenditure	10.42	11.01	11.65	13.91	15.92	17.94	16.6	16.76	5.66%	5.81%	36.65%	28.97%	-6.58%
Private insurance expenditure as a % of total expenditure	1.14	1.54	2.36	3.53	4.75	5.17	6.28	6.05	35.09%	53.25%	101.27%	46.46%	17.02%
Total household expenditure as a % of total expenditure	11.56	12.55	14.01	17.44	20.67	23.11	22.88	22.81	8.56%	11.63%	47.54%	32.51%	-1.30%
Real per capita public expenditure ($1,995)	1,309	1,252	1,417	1,404	1,383	1,353	1,379	1,395	-4.35%	13.18%	-2.40%	-3.63%	3.10%
Total expenditure as % of GDP	7.04	6.37	6.88	7.42	7.67	7.66	7.42	7.42	-9.52%	8.01%	11.48%	3.23%	-3.13%
Output statistics													
Waiting lists (no.)	39,848	42,972	56,175	62,638	65,240	76,577	74,806	85,624	7.84%	30.72%	16.14%	22.25%	11.81%
Public sector % daypatient*	9.9	10.6	15.6	14.2	19.3	NA	28.10	27.8	7.07%	47.17%	23.72%	NA	NA
Public sector average length of stay (days)**	7.6	7.5	7	6.5	6.2	NA	4.63	4.53	-1.32%	-6.67%	-11.43%	NA	NA
Public primary care expenditure*													
Benefits (not dental, maternity) ($000)	42,488	50,797	83,690	212,887	202,459	203,630	208,100	209,969	19.56%	64.75%	141.92%	-4.35%	3.11%
Maternity ($000)	7,077	11,091	35,290	58,936	67,248	78,222	89,618	89,594	56.72%	218.19%	90.56%	32.72%	14.54%
Referred Services ($000)****	26,467	43,308	75,192	110,847	110,210	119,223	135,419	146,046	63.63%	73.62%	46.57%	7.56%	22.50%
Pharmaceuticals ($000)	132,020	254,843	506,660	545,331	556,373	582,931	640,697	674,080	91.90%	98.81%	9.81%	6.89%	15.64%

All data year ended 30 June, unless otherwise stated. All data is GST inclusive: 10% from 1 October 1986; 12.5% from 1 July 1989.
Expenditure data is March years up to 1989; June years thereafter. Waiting list data is March years up to 1988; June years thereafter.
Sources: All expenditure data from Muthumala and Ellis (undated). Output statistics from McKendry et al. (undated) and Ministry of Health (1994/95).
* 1980–92 data is as % of total noncontinuing care patients; 1994 and 1995 data is % day surgery.
** 1980–92 data is average of stays less than 92 days; 1994 and 1995 data is case-mix adjusted.
*** Changes in contract arrangements from 1993 may reduce recorded expenditure in these categories.
**** Including specialist, laboratory and diagnostic imaging expenditures.
NA data not available; italicised data is 1982–83; bold data is 1984/85; Underlined data is from New Zealand Health Information Service, to March years.

increasingly funded by central government – have largely provided such services. These hospitals have traditionally been funded according to historical allocations, supplemented by payments for inflation and new services.

The voluntary (not for profit) sector has made major contributions to New Zealand health care, providing infant and child health; care for those with mental, intellectual and physical disabilities; and accommodation for the elderly. Succeeding governments have recognised this sector's importance by providing increasing levels of state funding.

The private sector, too, has played an important role in the delivery and financing of health care in New Zealand. Private practitioners are the dominant primary care providers, and while private hospitals have received government funding in the past, this has increasingly been limited to subsidies for long-stay care of the elderly. New Zealanders have also had access to supplementary private health insurance, with about a third of New Zealanders covered by private insurance by the early 1980s (Scott *et al.*, 1986). Such insurance allows faster access to elective care in private hospitals and covers the gap between government subsidies and primary care fees. However, private insurance has only ever contributed a small (but rapidly increasing) proportion of New Zealand's total health care costs.

These arrangements – particularly government control of hospital spending – have largely restrained growth in health care spending, and have provided at least the potential for good access to quality care for the entire population. Overall, New Zealand health policies have, however, been argued to be less successful at promoting incentives for technical efficiency and cost effectiveness in service delivery, while promoting fragmentation of service delivery, variations in access to services, a lack of accountability and a lack of planning and coordination (*A Health Service for New Zealand*, 1975; Scott *et al.*, 1986; Hospital and Related Services Taskforce, 1988).

In particular, subsidies in primary care have been available for only some categories of providers and services and have not always kept pace with practitioner fees, leading to rising levels of patient charges and perceived barriers to accessing care. Those living in rural areas have also faced difficulties in accessing primary care (Scott *et al.*, 1986). Further, the government has faced uncapped expenditure in primary care as a result of fee-for-service subsidies. In secondary care, increasing waiting lists and times for access to specialist assessments and treatment have become persistent problems since the 1960s (Hay, 1989). There have also been continuing difficulties in closing down and reducing the sophistication of services provided in small, largely rural, hospitals (Hay, 1989). In the voluntary sector, tensions have always existed between the desires of agencies to remain independent and policy makers' desires to improve coordination with other service delivery, improve accountability and ensure less variability in provision (*A Health Service for New Zealand*, 1975).

In terms of health status, New Zealanders have enjoyed internationally high levels of health, but this has fallen relative to a number of other countries since the 1960s (OECD, 1987). The health status of Maori (New Zealand's indigenous people) and children, in particular, has remained relatively poor (Pomare *et al.*, 1995).

External factors: economic and social policy reform in the 1980s and 1990s

Factors external to the health system affecting health reform in New Zealand mirror those which Moran has identified in this volume (Chapter 2). This is particularly true in relation to the rise of market ideologies in the search for increased competitiveness, and an emphasis on responsiveness to consumer needs, self-reliance and accountability. In the New Zealand case, economic and social policy reforms in the 1980s were related to poor economic performance from the late 1960s (Economic Monitoring Group, 1989) and pressure by influential interest groups and the main government advisor on economic and fiscal policy – The Treasury – for a more market, less interventionist, approach. With the election of the fourth Labour government in 1984, succeeding ministers of finance with a market-oriented approach proposed and oversaw implementation of a large number of economic and social policy reforms. In this they were aided by a unicameral system of government, elected under a first-past-the-post system, with overall policy control vested in a small group of cabinet ministers able to implement changes rapidly, despite significant public opposition.

Resulting economic and social policy reforms included deregulating markets and eliminating producer subsidies; restructuring government trading departments into profit-oriented enterprises and the later selling of such organisations to the private sector; introducing contractual arrangements between ministers and core government departments; flattening the income tax scale; moving towards increased targeting of state benefits to those on low incomes; and shifting the basis of funding voluntary organisations in health and social policy areas away from contracts for inputs to contracts for outputs. (For further information on New Zealand's economic and social policy reforms, see the Treasury, 1984, 1987; Easton, 1989; Boston and Dalziel, 1992; Smith, 1995; Kelsey, 1995; OECD, 1996.)

Health care reform in the 1980s

Reviews of the health sector were undertaken in 1975, 1986 and 1988 (*A Health Service for New Zealand*, 1975; Scott *et al.*, 1986; Hospital and Related Services Taskforce, 1988). Few recommendations arising from such reviews were implemented, due to professional and voluntary group opposition to contracting (Hay, 1989; Davies, 1990), and a lack of consensus on a direction for the sector.

Succeeding governments did, however, implement some reforms during the 1980s. The most significant reforms introduced population-based funding for publicly owned hospitals, and established 14 regionally based area health boards to take over responsibilities for purchasing and providing hospital and public health services. The fourth Labour government sought improved management and business approaches from area health boards by developing contract arrangements with boards and strengthening accountability to central government. This government also introduced user charges for pharmaceuticals and targeted increased government subsidies to those on lower incomes and with poorer health (Ashton, 1992). (The impact of these policies on public and private expenditures is set out in Table 7.1.)

At the same time, the increasing competence and organisation of consumer groups (particularly amongst women and Maori) brought increased pressure for reforms which would provide greater choice in service delivery and improve responsiveness to consumer needs and wants. In this vein, the Labour government was successful in passing legislation providing midwives with the ability to take responsibility for maternity care to the same level previously reserved for doctors, as well as access to fee-for-service subsidies. This occurred in spite of significant opposition from the medical profession.

Health reform proposals in 1991

The newly elected National government established a Health Services Taskforce in early 1991, sidestepping the usual advisory channels through the Department of Health. The government signalled the direction it desired from the outset. Objectives for the Taskforce made reference to focusing assistance 'on those least able to make provision for themselves', and the need for greater choice and competition between funders and between providers. In particular, the Taskforce was directed to consider whether a separation of funder and provider roles was required to promote competition among providers (Upton, 1991a).

Although the Taskforce drew on a range of international literature, the emphasis was on managed competition strategies, as promoted by Enthoven (1988), and on reforms proposed in the United Kingdom (Secretary of State for Health, 1989) and the Netherlands (Van de Ven, 1990). A number of people involved in the health sector in the United States and in reforms in the United Kingdom and the Netherlands visited New Zealand over the time the Taskforce met. The Taskforce drew on previous reports, Treasury documents (The Treasury, 1990a, 1990b) and a report commissioned by the New Zealand Business Roundtable (a private sector advocate of economic and social policy reforms along market lines) (Danzon and Begg, 1991), as well as the views of officials in various government departments. The Taskforce itself did not undertake any research on problems in the health sector, nor did it engage in any formal consultation on these problems or possible solutions.

The recommendations arising from Taskforce deliberations were released in the July 1991 budget. The reforms had the following objectives: improving access to services; improving efficiency, flexibility and innovation in the delivery of health care; widening choice and increasing the sensitivity of the sector to changing needs; enhancing the working environment for health professionals; and recognising the importance of public health in preventing illness and injury and in promoting health (Upton, 1991a). It was clear that the government expected decision making in health care to become less politicised (Upton, 1991a), while proposals for reform of social policy funding signalled the government's intentions to limit its role in funding health care (Shipley *et al.*, 1991).

Figure 7.1 sets out the structure of the reformed health sector as proposed in mid-1991. The main reform proposals were to:

- Split purchasing and provision functions of area health boards by establishing four regional health authorities (RHAs) as purchasing agents, and 23 Crown health enterprises (CHEs), to be run along business lines and to compete with private and voluntary organisations for contracts with RHAs.
- Integrate funding for primary and secondary care services, in order to enhance cost effectiveness and encourage better patient management and access to care.[2]
- Establish separate public health purchasing and provision agencies, in order to protect funding for population-based services.
- Allow, once RHAs and CHEs were established, individuals to opt out of their RHA and take a risk-adjusted premium to an alternative purchasing agent (health care plan), in order to provide a competitive incentive for RHAs to promote efficiency and responsiveness.
- Develop an explicit core of services to promote efficiency in competition between purchasing agents, accountability, improvements in equity of access and improved priority setting processes. Responsibility for defining the core would lie with an independent National Advisory Committee on Core Health Services.
- Introduce changes to the financing of health care. First, the government would target government subsidies to those on low incomes, increase user charges for pharmaceuticals and introduce new laboratory, hospital inpatient and outpatient charges. Second, the government set out options for the longer term financing of health care, as part of wider proposals for reform aimed at limiting government funding only to those on low incomes (Shipley *et al.*, 1991).

The government sought public and professional comment on only

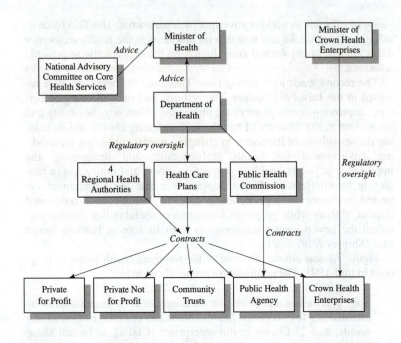

Figure 7.1 **The New Zealand health sector 1991 reform proposals**

two aspects of the reforms: the proposals for changes in the financing of health care, and how core services might be defined. All other reforms were planned to be implemented within two years, a timeframe which was to prove impossible.

Implementing the reforms

A significant outcry followed the announcement of the reform proposals, which were constantly in the media prior to and following the commencement of the new system. A number of consumer groups, academics and the public, as well as professional groups (nurses' organisations, GP groups, salaried specialists and a newly established Coalition for Public Health), voiced opposition to the reforms. Many objected to the lack of consultation on the proposals, and argued that the government could not therefore claim community support for them. Other contentious issues included the likely costs of the reforms, the loss of elected representatives in the reformed structure, fears that the government would sell publicly owned hospitals, although the Minister of Health denied this (Upton, 1991b), and concerns about the potential for the reforms to reduce access and equity of access. Some queried whether competition would develop in a small country with a geographically dispersed population, and suggested overall costs would rise because of undesirable quality competition, duplication in facilities, and overinvestment in expensive technology. Commentators argued that competition between purchasers would exacerbate such problems, leading to higher overall costs, and increased potential for cream skimming (for commentaries on the proposals see Ashton *et al.*, 1991; Powell, 1991; Bridgeport Group, 1992; Feek and Carter, 1992; Wellington Health Action Committee, 1992; Neutze, 1993).

At the same time, the magnitude and complexity of the reforms became more obvious. Implementation of the entire package required a significant amount of work by a number of new agencies established to oversee implementation, including: decisions on the structures of new institutions; policy work to unbundle and redistribute expenditure, and to develop an explicit core of services and formula to risk-rate premiums to fund RHAs and HCPs; and the establishment of new agencies and administrative systems to support reforms in the financing of health care. Even once the new agencies were in place, they would have major tasks to take on, including overall purchasing, business and contracting strategies; development of contract structures and documentation; collection and collation of existing and new service description, volume and comparable price data; and the development of relationships and negotiation of contract and incentive arrangements across the sector.

As National's political fortunes waned (Edwards, 1996) and the reforms became bogged down in implementation, the government dropped a number of proposals. It decided to retain tax-based financing of health care; to drop proposals for health care plans, following problems in developing methods to risk-rate health care premiums; to increase primary care subsidies for children; and to drop laboratory charges and inpatient charges in public hospitals. These decisions reduced the impact of user charges on consumer decisions, cemented continued government funding in place, and dismantled plans for competition in purchasing. A regional single purchaser model remained, with competition in provision the key market factor.

Further, in developing the legislation to underpin the reformed structure, the government was forced to consider the potential for market factors to generate unpopular outcomes (such as a closure of a facility, or changes in service availability). As a result, the government has placed requirements on RHAs to consult with their communities, in a system where RHAs are formally accountable to the government. Health legislation requires CHEs 'while operating as a successful and efficient business' to 'exhibit a sense of social responsibility by having regard to the interests of the community in which [it] operates' (Health and Disability Services Act, 1993, s. 11: 7–8). Legislation also provides ministerial powers to give direction to RHAs and to require CHEs to deliver particular services.

In the run-up to the start date of the reforms (1 July 1993) and the 1993 election, the government further slowed the pace of change. It announced a rollover of services delivered in 1992/93 and sought to ensure that CHEs received 98 per cent of their 1992/93 budgets in 1993/94 (Cooper, 1994). Further, in the light of significant opposition to contracts for primary care providers, the government provided RHAs with the ability to continue payments to providers without a formal contract, in effect allowing the continuation of fee-for-service payments for GPs and other professionals (Health and Disability Services Act, 1993, s.51).

Since the implementation of the modified reform structure in 1993, the government decided to integrate previously separate disability support funding into RHA budgets, abandoned plans to do the same with ACC payments, and reintegrated public health purchasing into RHA budgets. The government also handed over responsibility for pharmaceutical purchasing to the four RHAs in the form of a Pharmaceutical Management Company (Pharmac), owned by the four RHAs. The resulting structure, as of December 1996, is set out in Figure 7.2.

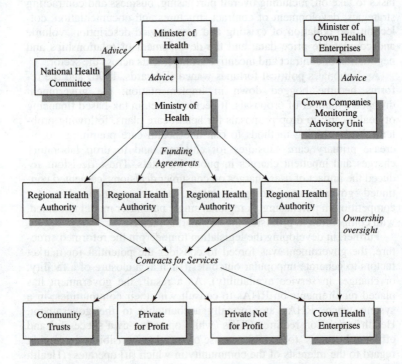

*Figure 7.2   **The New Zealand health and disability support sector 1996***

Analysis of the reform outcomes

In this section, we describe and analyse the reform outcomes, largely based on information available on the sector's performance to mid–1995. This analysis is, however, complicated by two main factors. First, very little research has been undertaken on the reforms. This has meant that a number of important issues are not able to be dealt with. For example, we make no attempt to analyse the effects of the reforms on the role and morale of professionals working in the sector.[3] Second, it is difficult to attribute all the changes occurring over the past few years to the reforms themselves because of a number of ongoing trends which predated the reforms and because of the government's allocation of an estimated additional $1.03 billion to RHAs between 1993 and mid–1996 (see Table 7.1 and McLoughlin, 1996). Many more millions have been provided to CHEs via debt write-offs and increases in government equity.

Effects on policy structures and processes

The funder–purchaser–provider split which forms the basis of the current health structure in New Zealand is potentially inefficient compared to a vertically integrated model, because of the impact of asset specificity, uncertainty, frequency of transactions and the measurability of attributes on transaction costs (Howden-Chapman and Ashton, 1994; Ashton, 1996). New Zealand's experiences to date are certainly suggestive of the type of problems that arise from such separation in the health sector, and are further complicated by the difficulties the government has had in removing itself from decision making in the sector.

First, there is confusion over the roles of the Minister and Ministry of Health and RHAs. RHAs are charged with assessing needs, consulting with their communities and ostensibly setting priorities, but a number of limits have developed around these roles. Funding allocated to personal health, disability support and public health can only be spent in those areas (called ring-fencing), while funding has also been increasingly tagged for spending on specific services (e.g. initiatives to reduce waiting times). Moreover, ministers of health have become involved in a number of major decisions relating to purchasing and service delivery, while also asking RHAs to meet a large number of requirements relating to service delivery, access and contracting (Howden-Chapman and Ashton, 1994; Office of the Minister of Health, 1996; Shipley, undated a). With so much decision making taking place at a central level, one wonders why RHAs exist at all.

Second, the reforms have highlighted difficulties in separating out responsibilities in purchasing and provision, fuelling arguments that such separation is undesirable and costly. For example, trade-offs must be made between contract specificity and flexibility for providers to allocate resources as health care needs and demands change. Some overlap of purchasing and provision is then inevitable. Further, suggestions have been made that providers require information about RHA purchasing strategies in order to develop business plans and set prices, and that CHEs find it difficult to invest in plant, equipment and service development when RHAs offer only short-term contracts. The current system also created early conflicts between CHE plans and RHA abilities to fund services, with poor communication between RHAs and those responsible for approving CHE business plans. A number of providers have also complained that RHAs have become involved in operating decisions (on these points, see Nahkies, 1995; Rivers Buchan Associates, 1995; Ministry of Health, undated).

Finally, tensions have arisen between CHE desires to make decisions on commercial principles and RHA and government desires to ensure continuity of service delivery, particularly where CHEs are monopoly providers. CHEs must therefore signal and consult on any intentions they may have to exit service provision, and the process of exiting services may then take a year or more to achieve (Nahkies, 1995; Ministry of Health, undated).

Contracting

Contracting arrangements play an important role in the reformed health sector, providing the mechanism through which RHAs can allocate resources, giving incentives to providers to meet sector objectives, and capping or better controlling previously uncapped expenditures.

Since 1993 the four RHAs have made significant progress towards developing contract arrangements with GPs. This is remarkable considering that such attempts have consistently failed in the past. By mid-1996, almost 20 per cent of GPs were on capitation contracts for general practice and other services, while 50 per cent of GPs were involved in budget-holding arrangements based around referred services (mainly pharmaceuticals and laboratory services) but not including payments for general practice services (personal communication, Performance Management Unit, Ministry of Health). Budgets are generally negotiated around historical expenditures, with GPs generally not carrying the risk of overexpenditure (Ministry of Health, 1994/95).

Developing contracting arrangements with CHEs has been one of the more difficult tasks in the sector. A review of contracting noted problems associated with long contract development times, a short one-year contract cycle, and poor communication between RHAs and providers. This review suggested that in 1994/95 negotiations with CHEs had not delivered benefits proportional to the time involved (Ministry of Health, undated). This situation may have improved slightly in 1995/96.

There have also been major concerns expressed about contracting for quality of care in the sector, particularly in relation to CHEs. A number of CHEs have viewed quality schedules in contracts as limited in their effects, and have argued that contract negotiations and prices do not reward quality (discussion at Health Services Research Centre Conference, 1995). This is an area which is just beginning to gain significant attention and where further work is urgently required.

The voluntary (not-for-profit) sector, too, has reported difficulties in contracting. They have experienced delays in concluding contracts, problems in planning service development with one-year contracts and problems with communication with RHAs (Rivers Buchan Associates, 1995).

Estimating the costs associated with contracting is problematic, due to the lack of baseline data and the difficulties in distinguishing between production and transaction costs (Ashton, 1996). A Ministry of Health review estimated RHA costs to be about $8 million or 0.2 per cent of funds allocated to RHAs for purchasing services.[4] CHEs estimated their costs at between $200,000 and $2 million plus. The Rest Homes Association has estimated its contracting costs at $1.8 million, and other providers also state that the costs they have incurred are quite high and in some cases, that costs are higher than under the previous system (Ministry of Health, undated; Ashton, 1996).

In spite of these problems, CHEs and voluntary providers have reported positive spin-offs from contracting processes, in particular from greater clarity and focus, and increased accountability (Rivers Buchan Associates, 1995; Ministry of Health, undated; Ashton, 1996).

Partly as a result of some of these issues, the existence of four RHAs continues to be a controversial issue. A review of the number of RHAs was undertaken in late 1994, with the Minister of Health deciding that four RHAs allowed for greater innovation and more relevant local and regional consultation. At the same time, the Minister recognised a number of concerns with early contracting strategies, and has suggested RHAs try to reduce transaction costs, for example by sharing information, developing common approaches to purchasing, developing longer term contracts, using simpler contracts for low-cost transactions, and combining related services into single contracts (Shipley, undated b).

Competition

In the New Zealand reforms, competition was expected to develop in two major ways. First, CHEs and private providers would compete on price and/or quality for contracts with RHAs. Second, competition was also expected to develop via more cost-effective ways of delivering services (e.g. nursing services, community care services).

Price and quality competition has not developed significantly in secondary care markets[5] (Ministry of Health, 1994/95; OECD, 1996), while a number of problems in developing more competitive markets have been reported. For example, prices sometimes rise as a result of competitive tendering, because CHE deficits continue to be subsidised by the government and CHEs sometimes seek to fully cost their services and add a further margin of around 5–10 per cent when tendering for additional contracts (Lovatt, 1996). Private sector prices have often been uncompetitive (Ministry of Health, undated; Wilson, 1995). Other issues have included concerns over potential discontinuities in service delivery (Foster, 1994; Ministry of Health, 1994/95; Lovatt, 1996), difficulties in specifying the services RHAs wish to buy with sufficient precision (OECD, 1996), and difficulties in defining the boundaries between contracts (Lovatt, 1996).

The reforms also implied that CHEs would be able to increase their revenues by expanding service delivery if they were able to deliver good quality services at a reasonable price. This has proved a largely elusive incentive, first because of equity concerns and secondly because of the slow development of quality audit and contracting on the basis of quality (see, e.g., Ashton, 1996). Where resources have been redistributed between CHEs this has been largely on the basis of aligning revenue with outputs (Wilson, 1995), and improving equity of access by contracting for rates of output (e.g. surgical operations per thousand population) closer to the (standardised) national average (Ministry of Health, 1994/95).

Competition in the form of benchmarking, particularly where the potential for competition appears limited, is often discussed among policy makers. Such competition is reliant on improving definitions and pricing methodologies (Ashby, 1996), but at the end of 1996 it remained unclear how far those in the sector expect competition to develop as compared to benchmarking approaches.

Competition was also expected to develop via more cost-effective ways of delivering services (e.g. nursing services, community care services). Beyond establishing some new contracts in primary care, progress in this area has been slow, although new opportunities for more cost-effective care are developing as budget-holding arrangements with GPs evolve. Increased interest is now being shown in the potential for such arrangements to develop into full budget-holding or managed care arrangements (perhaps incorporating budgets for secondary care services and with or without financial risk), and for other groups (such as Maori, nurses and community groups) to establish or become involved in managed care organisations.

Effects on efficiency

Any assessment of the effects of the reforms on efficiency is complicated by competing notions of efficiency. Ideally this section should focus on efficiency defined as improvements in health outcomes while maintaining or reducing costs across both private and public health expenditures (thereby incorporating notions of effectiveness, cost effectiveness and quality of care). However, most of the available information focuses largely on the volume and cost of outputs delivered in the sector, and it is this information which forms the basis for the discussion.

The reforms have been associated with an increased interest and emphasis on effectiveness, although this is not unique to New Zealand. The National Health Committee,[6] Pharmac, the RHAs and providers are increasingly considering effectiveness in their decision making (National Advisory Committee on Core Health and Disability Support Services, 1995; Pharmac, 1995; Working party for the 'Guidelines for Guidelines' initiative, 1996).

In a number of areas, the reforms have generated savings and/or led to reductions in the rate of growth of expenditures. For example, there have been a number of reports of savings arising from budget-holding activities, primarily in relation to pharmaceuticals and laboratory tests. An early Ministry of Health review of budget-holding arrangements found savings of between 1 and 18 per cent in pharmaceutical budgets, averaging 5 to 10 per cent of budgets (Ministry of Health, 1995). Kerr *et al.* (1996) have reported savings of 32.9 per cent and 20.7 per cent in pilot groups holding budgets for laboratory services (coupled with feedback, order form redesign and education) compared to a nonpilot group's savings of 20.3 per cent. In addition, the overall performance of these three groups led to savings of almost 17 per cent compared to national cost increases of around 7 per cent.

Savings made from such initiatives have been used to cover contract and information systems costs (estimated at between $30,000 and $600,000), but also to improve access to care and develop new services (Ministry of Health, 1994/95).

The extent of the savings, however, is very much dependent on the ways in which the budgets are actually set in the first place. In addition, there is little evidence on the impact of these arrangements on quality of care and it is still too early to identify any effects on health status. Further, no research has been undertaken to suggest whether the costs involved in negotiating these arrangements have been worth the benefits generated.

Pharmac has made considerable savings in the past few years. Using a reference price scheme which sets a full government subsidy for only the lowest price drug in any therapeutic subgroup and contract arrangements to shift the risk of increased expenditures onto suppliers, Pharmac has been able to reduce the rate of growth of pharmaceutical expenditure from around 10 per cent per annum to 5 per cent per annum (Pharmac, 1995). Once again, the impact of these policies on patient costs and access and health outcomes has not been evaluated.

In secondary care, there are examples where competition has enabled increased outputs and reduced waiting times. Foster (1994) reported savings of around $300,000 and $365,000 for 1993/94 and 1994/95 respectively as a result of tendering. Hoskins *et al.* (1996) have reported on a joint private venture/CHE initiative which reduced waiting times and increased the numbers of patients treated (although readmissions increased). Lovatt (1996) notes that tendering has allowed shortened waiting times for some services for residents in the Midland region.

In promoting the reforms, the Minister of Health suggested that CHEs would make significant efficiency gains, partly as a result of increasing management flexibility, and partly due to improved incentives (Upton, 1991a). A Ministry of Health review stated that to mid-1995 overall efficiency in CHEs did not appear to have improved: additional outputs from the sector match the additional resources made available to CHEs after adjustment for inflation (Ministry of Health, 1994/95).

On other measures, CHE performance has not improved significantly over area health board performance prior to the reforms: trends in both length of stay and in day patient attendances have stabilised (McKendry *et al.*, undated; Ministry of Health, 1994/95; Ashby, 1996 and see Table 7.1), while costs appear to have increased faster than under the previous area health boards (Ashby, 1996).

The overall impact of the reforms on CHE efficiency remains, unclear, however, particularly as quality of care is not well measured and because of the necessity for CHEs to spend resources on much-needed maintenance and investment (following a run down of capital in the 1980s) and on management and information systems. In addition, the need to focus attention on collecting and interpreting information on services, volumes and prices appears to have taken a great deal more time than was expected. The jury is therefore still out in relation to the effects of the reforms and contracting on CHE performance.

Equity effects

A key objective of the reform process was to redistribute funding and services to improve access to care in some localities and reduce perceived overservicing in others. Some important achievements have been made towards this objective. A significant amount of activity is enabling better and new services to be delivered to Maori. RHAs have been developing copurchasing strategies with Maori, contracting with CHEs and other providers for improvements in cultural appropriateness, promoting Maori programmes and providing facilitation for Maori providers (Ministry of Health, 1994/95). It is still too early to identify significant gains in health status or measured gains in access to services for Maori, but the future here looks promising.

In primary care, RHAs appear to be aiming towards improved equity of access through identification of service gaps and the purchasing of additional primary care services. For example, in Coromandel, Midland RHA has purchased free GP care for children under five in order to improve access to care, and new services are being developed for young people and in mental health (Ministry of Health, 1994/95).

But funding arrangements for primary care continue to be based largely around historical expenditures, even where budget-holding arrangements are being implemented. In the short term, this policy will not remove longstanding inequities in levels of expenditures between communities (Malcolm, 1996). RHAs are now beginning to seek ways of limiting the number of GPs in areas regarded as overserviced, possibly by refusing to allow access to subsidies for GPs trained elsewhere ('Section 51 ruling still being sought', 1996). Many GPs support workforce management (Tyler, 1996), but at this stage the policies RHAs will use to achieve this goal remain unclear.

In secondary care, variations in access generally continue. The government and purchasers have, however, sought improved equity by contracting for surgical rates of intervention at the (standardised) national average (Ministry of Health, 1994/95). This approach is somewhat unsatisfactory, as there is no clear evidence that the national average is an appropriate level of care, or that differences in intervention rates are not in some way related to different levels of needs. This issue is now being addressed by the development of priority criteria and booking systems (see below).

Reconfiguration of services

The reforms have yet to show significant benefits from a reconfiguration of services (e.g. improving access and cost effectiveness by shifting services into the community, and improving coordination of care).

The integration of funding for primary, secondary and disability support services has been an important step in attempting to reconfigure services. In practice, ring-fencing arrangements around various categories of expenditure may reduce RHAs' ability to reconfigure services, while RHAs initially have also been unable to shift resources from CHEs to spend elsewhere (Ministry of Health, 1994/95).

Examples of services being reconfigured are particularly prominent for services for people with intellectual and psychiatric disabilities, although these policies predated the reforms. Attempts have also been made to improve the coordination of maternity care (and better control costs) by developing arrangements around a lead maternity provider, who will take overall responsibility for a woman's maternity and postnatal care. RHAs, GPs and midwives remained deadlocked over these arrangements for some time, although in Wellington new contract arrangements were put in place by September 1996 (Swain, 1996).

The status of small, largely rural, hospitals has been a perennial policy issue in New Zealand, particularly when it comes to their role in delivering surgical services. Although RHAs have faced continued opposition to changes in rural hospital status, in some cases they have been able to improve access to low-intensity services such as emergency and stabilisation care, day surgery and specialist assessments, at the same time as reducing the volumes of more intensive services delivered (North Health, 1995; Midland Health, 1995; Southern RHA, 1994/95).

Effects on users

This section considers the effects of the reforms on health care consumers using three areas of information: consumer satisfaction with CHE services, the numbers of services delivered and waiting lists and times.

Crown Companies Monitoring Advisory Unit survey data from CHEs generally show an increase in consumer satisfaction between mid-1993 and June 1995 over all CHEs, although individual CHE performance is variable. As perceptions of CHE performance are likely to be affected by factors other than the care provided (e.g. media attention to adverse events), these measures must be treated with some caution (Crown Companies Monitoring Advisory Unit unpublished data). The number of patients treated continues to increase generally across the publicly funded sector (Ministry of Health, 1994/95; Muthumala and Ellis, undated). Given the additional resources made available to the sector, the impact of the reforms themselves remain difficult to estimate, however. Between March 1993 and March 1995, waiting lists increased by 11.8 per cent to 85,624, and have increased further by 11.5 per cent to 95,470 by March 1996 (NZHIS data, Ministry of Health; see also Table 7.1). In terms of waiting times, aggregate data on the number of months required to clear waiting lists show some stability, at seven months in 1991 (McKendry *et al.*, undated), 6.1 months in 1993/94, and 6.8 months in 1994/95 (Ministry of Health, 1994/95).[8] Data from *Consumer* surveys in 1993 and 1995 show no significant change in waiting times, except for a deterioration in the proportion of patients seeing their specialist within three months of referral from 80 per cent to 76 per cent (Consumers' Institute 1995)[9]. These experiences are confirmed by RHA and CHE data on waiting times, although in some specialities waiting times have fallen considerably (Ministry of Health, 1994/95).

More recently, the government has announced the implementation of a booking system, by which elective patients will be assessed against priority criteria, and allocated a booked time for treatment within six months of assessment if they score a certain number of clinical points (Office of the Minister of Health, 1996). This system will increase the certainty of treatment for patients who meet the relevant clinical score and who previously may have languished on waiting lists without knowledge of whether or when they might be treated, and make the rationing of public health care resources in New Zealand much more explicit.

Discussion

In aiming to reform New Zealand's health sector, the government tried to shock the health system into reform and into a totally new structure. The complexities of establishing the new structures and collating the information to run it, and the government's failure to obtain significant support for the reforms, has meant that the government has been unable to implement the reforms as originally intended. In addition, the government has had to make political concessions by managing the role of the market in the sector and providing significant additional resources for health care.

To date, it appears unlikely that the benefits of the reforms have been worth the costs incurred. The benefits achieved to date have been limited, but include: the development of contract arrangements with primary care providers, better management of pharmaceutical costs, increased service options for Maori and the reconfiguration of some rural services. There are also signs of increased innovation, an increased interest in effectiveness and a potential for improved cost effectiveness and coordination of care arising from budget-holding and managed care arrangements. Improved accountability and information systems have also resulted from the reforms.

The costs associated with the reforms remain unquantified, but they are likely to have included quite high one-off transition costs associated with a settling in period for the new sector and a focus on collecting information (particularly in CHEs) – in all likelihood leading to a slow-down in the rate of change compared with the previous structure – and costs associated with the agencies established to implement the reforms. New information requirements (particularly in CHEs) are also likely to be costly, although the sector could not continue to operate efficiently without some new investment in this area. The reformed sector very likely incurs higher ongoing costs associated with new structures and the costs that providers now incur in contracting. The ongoing extent of these costs depends very much on whether the sector moves towards relational contracting arrangements (Ashton, 1996), and better coordination and sharing of information between agencies in the sector. The extent to which this will happen is not yet clear.

Such an analysis, however, provides a static view of the effect of the reforms on health sector performance. As the OECD noted in a recent report (1996:117), 'It is too early to observe [the reforms'] effects on health outcomes and also to discern what impact they will ultimately have on the outpus of the health sector ... '.

So what of the future? Much is made of the potential for the new structure to encourage the development of managed care arrangements, which may allow better integration of primary and secondary care and improved cost effectiveness. Yet RHAs may find it difficult to encourage further reconfiguration of services, particularly as any attempts to reduce CHE services may run up against public concern at any shift of services away from CHEs. Furthermore, significant policy work is required if primary care budgets are to be capped or managed care is to develop further. For example, there is a need to develop a risk-adjusted formula to fund managed care organisations equitably; to manage the redistribution of funding in any move away from historical to population-based funding; and to develop careful monitoring arrangements to ensure providers do not engage in cream skimming or cost-shifting behaviour, and that quality of care is not adversely affected.

It is also clear that the government continues to see a role for competitive tendering in the sector (Shipley, undated b). New Zealand's experiences suggest that competition in hospital sector provision is taking some time to develop and there is as yet no clear indication of how far competition in the secondary care sector might develop before the costs associated with possible duplication of facilities, loss of economies of scale and scope, and coordination begin to outweigh any benefits.

There are also signs that competition in purchasing may eventually emerge,[10] particularly if developing managed care organisations are encouraged to compete for patient registrations. The future of RHAs then becomes somewhat uncertain. One possible scenario is for RHAs to play a role similar to that of the 'alliances' proposed in United States reform (e.g. providing information on plan services and quality, monitoring of plan behaviour and outcomes, overseeing marketing) (White, 1995). As commentators on the original reform proposals noted, however, the benefits associated with managed competition are uncertain and the risks in terms of overall costs and the potential impact on equity are high (Ashton *et al.*, 1991; Powell, 1991; Bridgeport Group, 1992; Feek and Carter, 1992; Wellington Health Action Committee, 1992; Neutze, 1993; see also White, 1995).

In the meantime, there is an increased likelihood of very different arrangements developing around the country. The reforms have been successful in allowing more innovation in provision, but it is important for differing approaches to be carefully evaluated if we are to encourage successful models. There are no signs of concerted efforts to carry out such evaluations, while New Zealand continues to have no nationally organised and funded research and development strategy.

Of equal importance is that issues around the future of financing health care in New Zealand remain unresolved. Even in late 1996, real per capita public expenditure has not returned to the level of 1989/90 (Table 7.1), while an estimated 40–50 per cent of New Zealanders now have private supplementary health insurance (Consumers' Institute, 1995). Government statements are that funding for the sector will increase only in relation to changes in the composition and size of New Zealand's population (Shipley, undated a). This is unlikely to prove a sustainable policy, given continued pressure in the sector from an ageing population, new technologies, increasing expectations, continuing uncapped primary care budgets and constant pressure to increase funding for elective surgery. The role of patient fees in accessing primary care also remains an issue in New Zealand as such fees are a potential barrier to access. In addition, the new system continues to provide incentives to shift costs towards the private sector (e.g as may be occurring in pharmaceuticals and minor elective surgery). With private insurance costs rising (Bailey, 1996), government policies must turn their attention to overall health costs if they are to promote reasonable equity of access to care and to prevent cost blowouts occurring in a largely unregulated private insurance sector.

In the run-up to the October 1996 election, health was a key election issue and the reforms remain unpopular with the public (McLoughlin, 1996). A number of opposition parties argued for a return to aspects of the prereform health structure, including integration of purchasing and provision or a reduction in the number of RHAs, the removal of commercial incentives for hospitals, protection for rural hospitals and a return to elected area health boards (Pemble, 1996).

Overall, the reforms have remained controversial and the future of the structure looks shaky. Even if the architects of the reforms gain power following the 1996 election, pressure may come on them to justify the current structures or return to earlier models. As we have shown, the government has little that it can identify to suggest that these reforms have to date been worth the effort and costs involved. However, the problems about which people are concerned existed long before the governments of the 1980s and 1990s sought to address them, and although there is no certainty yet that the new structure will alleviate these problems, when the sector's original problems are considered, there is also nothing to suggest that a return to the past will prove a better solution.

Postscript

In December 1996, a National Party–New Zealand First coalition government announced new policy proposals for the health sector. These proposals emphasise the government role in funding and providing health services, and cooperation and collaboration rather than competition. Although the policy retains the purchaser–provider split, the four RHAs are to be replaced by a single funding body separate from the Ministry of Health. CHEs will be required to function in a businesslike manner, their competitive profit focus will be removed, and they will be reformed into an as-yet-unknown number of regional hospital and community services, with a focus on achieving health outcomes and improving the health status of the population they serve. The policy also appears to limit the potential for private providers to deliver services usually provided by the public sector, while GP budget-holding beyond subsidies for GP services, pharmaceuticals and laboratory services must be approved by the Minister of Health. Elected community representation in the reformed system is to be considered by a working party. Additional funding is to be provided over the next three years for (amongst other things) elective hospital treatment, the removal of hospital user charges, Maori provider development, mental health services and to provide for free doctor's visits and prescription medicines for children under five years of age.

At the time of writing, these policy proposals remained undeveloped. It is therefore difficult to evaluate the extent to which the integrity of the purchaser–provider split will remain, and the extent to which competitive features and the role of the private sector in health care will develop in future. It is also unclear how far the new regional and community services will resemble area health boards, and how the government intends to continue moves towards greater integration of services for primary, secondary, public health and disability care.

Notes

1. Additional arrangements existed for disability support services, public health and for accident-related care (known as ACC). This chapter does not discuss arrangements and reforms in these areas, nor in mental health, in detail.
2. ACC payments were also to be integrated into RHA budgets over time.
3. Poor morale may be a particular problem in CHEs (Brett, 1996; Coalition for Public Health, 1996). As poor morale was also argued to be a feature of the previous structure (Hospital and Related Services Taskforce, 1988; Upton, 1991a), not all of these problems are necessarily related to the 1991 reforms.
4. These costs did not include other costs associated with purchasing, such as needs analysis or decisions to buy particular services (Ministry of Health, undated).
5. Purchasers have been able successfully to employ competitive incentives to reduce prices in continuing care and mental health services, where a number of alternative private providers existed prior to the reforms.
6. This Committee, formerly called the National Advisory Committee on Core Health and Disability Support Services, was originally established to define an explicit core of services. It has moved away from this task. (For more information, see Cumming, 1994.)
7. Although waiting lists are not a good indicator of performance in the health sector, the data on waiting lists is reported here because the government placed a great deal of emphasis on long waiting lists as a signal that the prereform health structure was not working well. As a result, data on waiting lists have been used extensively in criticisms of the reforms and have therefore been a

powerful political influence in the sector in the past few years. The ability of the sector to deliver elective services has, however, been compromised by rising levels of acute services (Ministry of Health, 1994/95).

8. These data are not well developed, as they do not represent a consistent approach to placing people on or reviewing waiting lists across the country.

9. These surveys are of Consumers' Institute membership, who are slightly older and wealthier than the New Zealand population.

10. In the immediate future, ACC will also purchase services from CHEs and other providers, thereby introducing a degree of competition in purchasing.

References

Ashby, M. (1996) 'Performance improvement in the health sector'. Paper presented at the 1996 conference of the New Zealand Institute of Health Management, October.

Ashton, T. (1992) 'Reform of the health services: Weighing up the costs and benefits', in J. Boston and P. Dalziel (eds) *The Decent Society*, Auckland: Oxford University Press.

Ashton, T. (1996) 'Contracting for health services in New Zealand: Early experiences'. Paper presented at the International Health Economics Association Inaugural Conference, May 19–23.

Ashton, T., Beasley, D., Alley, P. and Taylor, G. (1991) *Reforming the New Zealand Health System: Lessons from Other Countries*, Auckland: Report of a study tour sponsored by Health Boards New Zealand.

Bailey, G. (1996) 'Health insurance costs jump by up to 20pc', *The Evening Post*, 6 August: 1.

Boston, J. and Dalziel, P. (eds) (1992) *The Decent Society*, Auckland: Oxford University Press.

Brett, C. (1996) 'Clash of the codes: Anarchy at Christchurch hospital', *North and South*, August: 86–94.

Bridgeport Group (1992) *The Core Debate: Stage One: How We Define the Core: Review of Submissions*, Wellington: Department of Health.

Coalition for Public Health (1996) *Rebuilding the Public Health System: Proposals for a New Health Policy*, Wellington: Coalition for Public Health.

Consumers' Institute (1995) 'Sick health?', *Consumer*, **338**: 23–5.

Cooper, M. (1994) 'Jumping on the spot – health reform New Zealand style', *Health Economics*, **3**: 69–72.

Cumming, J. (1994) 'Core services and priority setting: The New Zealand experience', *Health Policy*, **29** (1/2): 41–60.

Danzon, P. and Begg, S. (1991) *Options for Health Care in New Zealand*, Wellington: New Zealand Business Roundtable.

Davies, G. (1990) 'New Zealand health care: From ossification to action', *The Journal of Health Administration Education*, **8** (3): 367–89.

Easton, B. (ed) (1989) *The Making of Rogernomics*, Auckland: Auckland University Press.

Economic Monitoring Group (1989) *The Economy in Transition: Restructuring to 1989*, Wellington: New Zealand Planning Council.

Edwards, B. (1996) 'Steaming toward the MMP horizon', *The Evening Post*, September 7: 9.

Enthoven, A. (1988) *Theory and Practice of Managed Competition in Health Care Finance, Lectures in economics, theory, institutions, policy: G*, Amsterdam: Elsevier.

Feek, C. and Carter, J. (1992) 'Look before you leap – your health and the public health. State or market?', *New Zealand Medical Journal*, **105**: 294–6.

Foster, G. (1994) 'Gains from tendering elective surgery', *Health Manager*, **1** (3): 9–10.

Hay, I. (1989) *The Caring Commodity: The Provision of Health Care in New Zealand*, Auckland: Oxford University Press.

Health and Disability Services Act 1993, Wellington: New Zealand Government.

A Health Service for New Zealand (1975) Wellington: Government Printer.

Hoskins, R., Blaxall, M. and Sceats, J. (1996) *Venturo: Evaluation of a Pilot Specialist Budget-holding Contract: Report on the First Two Years*, Midland Health and Disability Analysis Unit Evaluation Series Number 1, Hamilton: Midland Health.

Hospital and Related Services Taskforce (1988) *Unshackling the Hospitals*, Wellington: Hospital and Related Services Taskforce.

Howden-Chapman, P. and Ashton, T. (1994) 'Shopping for health: Purchasing health services through contracts', *Health Policy*, **29** (1/2): 61–83.

Kelsey, J. (1995) *The New Zealand Experiment: A World Model for Structural Adjustment?*, Auckland: Auckland University Press with Bridget Williams Books.

Kerr, D., Malcolm, L., Schousboe, J. and Pimm, F. (1996) 'Successful implementation of laboratory budget holding by Pegasus Medical Group', *New Zealand Medical Journal*, **109**: 334–7.

Lovatt, D. (1996) 'Lessons from contestability', *Health Manager*, **3** (1): 12–15.

Malcolm, L. (1996) 'Inequities in access to and utilisation of primary medical care services for Maori and low income New Zealanders'. Paper presented at the Managed Care Conference, Auckland, May.

McKendry, C.G., Howard, P.S. and Carryer, B.E. (undated) *New Zealand Hospital Sector Performance 1983–1992*, Wellington: Performance Monitoring and Review Section, Ministry of Health.

McLoughlin, D. (1996) 'How bad is our health: Is New Zealand's number one concern beyond solving?', *North and South*, August: 69–77.

Midland Health (1995) *Annual Report 1995*, Hamilton: Midland Health.

Ministry of Health (1994/95) *Purchasing for Your Health: 1994/95*, Wellington: Contract Monitoring, Ministry of Health.

Ministry of Health (1995) *Descriptive Review of Selected Primary Health Care Initiatives*, Wellington: Ministry of Health.

Ministry of Health (undated) *Review of 1994/95 RHA contracting*, Wellington: Performance Monitoring and Review, Ministry of Health.

Muthumala, D. and Ellis, J.A. (undated) *Health Expenditure Trends in New Zealand 1980–1995*, Wellington: Sector Analysis Section, Ministry of Health.

Nahkies, G. (1995) 'Health sector contracting – a progress report from a provider perspective', *Public Sector*, **18** (1): 15–17.

National Advisory Committee on Core Health and Disability Support Services

(1995) *Fourth Annual Report*, Wellington: National Advisory Committee on Core Health and Disability Support Services.

Neutze, J. (1993) 'Health reforms and the public hospitals', *New Zealand Medical Journal*, **106**: 17–18.

North Health (1995) *Annual Report 1995*, Auckland: North Health.

OECD (1996) *New Zealand 1996*, OECD Economic Surveys, Paris: OECD.

OECD (1987) *Financing and Delivering Health Care: A Comparative Analysis of OECD Countries*, OECD Social Policy Studies, No. 4, Paris: OECD.

Office of the Minister of Health (1996) 'Media release: Funding boost to tackle waiting lists', Wellington: Minister of Health.

Pemble, L. (1996) 'Policies lack strategy', *New Zealand Doctor*, 21 August: 23–5.

Pharmac (1995) *Annual Review for the Year Ended 30 June 1995*, Wellington: Pharmac.

Pomare, E., Keefe-Orsmby, V., Ormsby, C., Pearce, N., Reid, P., Robson, B. and Watene-Haydon, N. (1995) *Hauora: Maori Standards of Health III: A Study of the Years 1970–1991*, Wellington: Te Ropu Rangahau Hauora a Eru Pomare.

Powell, I. (1991) 'And a sceptical view', *New Zealand Medical Association Newsletter* in *New Zealand Medical Journal*, **104**: 5.

Rivers Buchan Associates (1995) *RHAs Don't Fund: They Purchase Services*, Wellington: NZ Federation of Voluntary Welfare Organisations.

Scott, C., Fougere, G. and Marwick, J. (1986) *Choices for Health Care*, Wellington: Health Benefits Review.

Secretary of State for Health (1989) *Working for Patients*, London: HMSO.

'Section 51 ruling still being sought' (1996), *GP Weekly*, 21 August: 2.

Shipley Hon. J. (undated a) *Policy Guidelines for Regional health authorities 1996/97*, Wellington: Minister of Health.

Shipley, Hon. J. (undated b) *Advancing Health in New Zealand*, Wellington: Minister of Health.

Shipley, Hon. J. with Upton, S., Smith, L. and Luxton, J. (1991) *Social Assistance: Welfare that Works: A Statement of Government Policy on Social Assistance*, Wellington: Minister of Social Welfare.

Smith, V. (1995) *Contracting for Social and Welfare Services: The Changing Relationship between Government and the Voluntary Sector*, MPP Research Paper, Victoria University of Wellington.

Southern Regional Health Authority (1994/95) *1994/95 Annual Report*, Dunedin: Southern Regional Health Authority.

Swain, P. (1996) 'Birth without the tantrums', *The Dominion*, September 2: 9.

The Treasury (1984) *Economic Management*, Wellington: The Treasury.

The Treasury (1987) *Government Management*, Wellington: The Treasury.

The Treasury (1990a) *Briefing to the Incoming Government 1990*, Wellington: The Treasury.

The Treasury (1990b) *Performance of the Health System*, Report to the Minister of Finance, Wellington: The Treasury.

Tyler, V. (1996) 'Workforce regulation gets big tick – GPA survey', *GP Weekly*, 10 April: 1.

Upton, S. (1991a) *Your Health and the Public Health: A Statement of Government Health Policy*, Wellington: Minister of Health.

Upton (1991b) quoted in 'A letter from the Minister', *New Zealand Medical Association Newsletter* in *New Zealand Medical Journal*, **104**: 2.

Van de Ven, W. (1990) 'From regulated cartel to regulated competition in the Dutch health care system', *European Economic Review*, **34**: 632–45.

Wellington Health Action Committee (1992) *Health Reforms: A Second Opinion*, Wellington: Wellington Health Action Committee.

White, J. (1995) *Competing Solutions: American Health Care Proposals and International Experience*, Washington DC: Brookings Institution.

Wilson, G. (1995) 'Health purchasing: A regional health authority perspective', *Public Sector*, **18** (1): 11–14.

Working party for 'Guidelines for Guidelines' initiative (1996) *Guidelines for Guidelines* (draft), Auckland: Working party for 'Guidelines for Guidelines' initiative.

Acknowledgements

The authors would like to thank the numerous people who made comments on earlier versions of this paper. We gratefully acknowledge the funding of the Health Research Council of New Zealand in undertaking the research for this paper. The views expressed are, however, those of the authors alone.

CHAPTER 8

Managed competition: health care reform in the Netherlands

RAY ROBINSON

Introduction

The Netherlands provides a fascinating case study for anyone interested in the role of competition policy in health care reform. The proposals, as set out in the Dekker Report (1987) under the title 'Willingness to Change', represent (from a mainstream economics perspective) probably the most comprehensive and coherent approach to managed competition to be found among the many national examples of health care reform. The main elements of the programme are based upon both demand and supply-side competition within a managed or regulatory framework. It is significant that a major study of health care reforms in 12 countries carried out by National Economic Research Associates (NERA) – which sought to produce a prototype for international reform combining the efficiency gains from competition with an equity objective ensuring universal access to health care for the whole population – based its proposals on those put forward in the Netherlands (Hoffmeyer and McCarthy, 1994; Towse, 1995).

However, as Moran has pointed out in Chapter 2, it would be a mistake to view the process of health care reform solely in terms of the coherence of its economic components. The imperatives for reform, and the direction that reform takes in any country, depend upon the complex interplay of numerous economic, social and political factors. These factors have been particularly apparent in the Netherlands in relation to the progress, or lack of it, in implementing the Dekker proposals.

In this chapter an attempt is made to bring together a discussion of these economic, political and social considerations. The main elements of the Dutch reform proposals are described, followed by an analysis of some of the key aspects of the proposals. Then an account of events following the publication of the proposals is presented together with a consideration of those factors that have determined the pace of change. The final section reflects upon the role of competition policy within Dutch society. Before embarking on this account, however, the next section outlines the main features of the health care system as it existed in the Netherlands at the time of the reform proposals, and of the factors that led to calls for reform.

The health care system in the Netherlands

This section examines the main features of the Dutch health care system in terms of the sources and methods of finance, and the organisation, incentives and behaviour of providers in the primary and secondary care sectors.

Health finance

The cultural belief underpinning the Dutch health care system combines a strong commitment to social solidarity with a simultaneous concern with individualism. The commitment to social solidarity results in a belief that health care should be funded collectively on the basis of ability to pay and that access should be based upon levels of patient needs. At the same time, support for individualism means that emphasis is placed upon obligations rather than rights, and leads to a concern with the way that the health care sector is bound together by mutual, interlocking obligations (Kirkman-Liff, 1991; Kirkman-Liff and Maarse, 1992). The health finance system endeavours to embody both of these values. It comprises compulsory social insurance, together with discretionary private insurance.

Compulsory social insurance is provided under two pieces of legislation. First, there is the Exceptional Medical Expenses Act (AWBZ) which came into force in 1967 (Ministry of Welfare, Health and Cultural Affairs, 1989). Initially, this Act covered long-term and high cost care, but over the years its scope has been extended. In recent years the services it has covered include long-term hospital care, nursing home care, residential care for people with learning disabilities, vaccinations, day care in nursing homes, psychiatric outpatient and nonresidential care and medicines. Insurance under the Act is compulsory with practically the whole of the population making income-related contributions together with a smaller flat rate payment.

Alongside AWBZ there is the Health Insurance Act which came into force in 1966. This Act offers coverage for basic medical care and is compulsory for approximately two-thirds of the population whose incomes fall below a specified ceiling. People covered by the scheme are required to make income-related payments together with smaller flat rate charges. Employers are also required to make payments on behalf of their employees. Services covered under the Health Insurance Act include: treatment by GPs, hospital care, dental care, and various specialised services such as audiology, haemodialysis and services for patients with chronic respiratory disease.

Contributions made under the Exceptional Medical Expenses Act and the Health Insurance Act are administered by the Central Sickness Fund Council (*Ziekenfondsraad*) which makes payments to individual sickness funds. The council has 37 members drawn from government, providers of medical care, individual sickness funds, employers and employees as well as representatives of consumers and patients' associations. The individual sickness funds are not-for-profit, originally regionally based organisations, often with charitable origins. They are responsible for making payments on behalf of patients to health care providers. In the late 1980s there were over 40 regional sickness funds but since then they have been the subject of considerable rationalisation and amalgamation. Today about 60 per cent of the population is enrolled in approximately 25 sickness funds operating nationwide (Okma, 1995). It is expected that eventually there will probably be only between 10 and 15 funds remaining (Van de Ven and Rutten, 1994).

Most of the one-third of the population whose incomes are above the eligibility level for coverage under the Health Insurance Act take out private insurance with one of the 40 or more private insurers. Approximately 60 per cent of private insurance is in the form of individual contracts, with the remainder on a group contract basis.

Although the private insurance industry serves that section of the population not eligible for coverage under the Health Insurance Act, there is a good deal of collaboration with the not-for-profit sickness funds. In fact, the largest private insurance company, Silver Cross, which has over 600,000 subscribers, was originally founded in 1948 following an initiative on the part of the sickness funds. At the time the funds were concerned about the problems facing their members when their incomes rose above the ceiling level making them ineligible for insurance by the funds. In response to this situation, Silver Cross was developed with the aim of offering high quality services at affordable premium levels.

Health providers: primary health care

The Netherlands has an extensive system of primary health care based upon approximately 7,000 general practice (GP) doctors and a further 7,000 community nurses (Okma, 1995, Hoffmeyer and McCarthy, 1994). Dutch GPs work as independent contractors for the sickness funds and private insurers in much the same way as British GPs work with the NHS. More than half the GPs work as single-handed practices, while about 40 per cent are in small partnerships. A limited number of GPs (less than 10 per cent) work in health centres alongside community nurses and social workers.

Under the provisions of the Health Insurance Act, patients may register with a GP of their choice and the GP receives a capitation payment for each registered patient. Patients covered by private insurance generally pay their GPs a fee-for-service per consultation. In the publicly funded sector, access to secondary care is controlled through GP referrals. Similarly, most private insurers require a GP referral before access to specialist services is authorised. Thus, GPs in the Netherlands are in a strong position to act as gatekeepers to secondary care.

Care is also provided in primary or community settings by community nurses. The service is organised on a national basis through regional organisations and local teams, with each local team comprising around 10 nurses. These nurses concentrate upon child health care and nursing care for the elderly. Patients have direct access to community nursing which is insured under AWBZ.

Health care providers: the hospital sector

Many social institutions in the Netherlands have been developed on either a religious (Catholic or Protestant) or a political (Socialist or Liberal) basis. These have been described as the 'four pillars' of Dutch society, each seeking to maintain its distinctive cultural identity (Saltman and de Roo, 1989). The hospital sector reflects this emphasis, with the majority of the country's hospitals retaining a religious character.

All of these hospitals are owned and operated on a not-for-profit basis by private, locally controlled, independent boards. In fact, private for-profit hospitals are prohibited by law. Traditionally most hospital specialists worked as independent practitioners and were paid on a fee-for-service basis. However, in recent years, there has been a rapid move towards salaried medical specialists so that they currently represent approximately 50 per cent of the profession.

During the 1980s, government policy encouraged a series of mergers between hospitals in the belief that this would reap economies of scale and lead to reductions in excess capacity. However, this policy led to criticisms that it was likely to stifle competition (Schut *et al.*, 1991) and was abandoned in the early 1990s.

Government policy has also sought to contain the rate of increase in hospital costs through changes in the financial arrangements governing hospital behaviour. Until 1983, hospitals received full retrospective payment for all of the services they provided. Combined with the fee-for-service system through which doctors were paid, this provided a strong incentive to maximise the number of inpatient days. The result was both high admission rates and long lengths of stay.

In an effort to address this problem, a new system of prospective global budgeting was introduced in 1983. Under this arrangement, hospitals received a fixed budget allocation for the financial year ahead. Because any overspends would need to be met from within the hospitals' own resources it was hoped that this system would offer stronger incentives for cost containment (Maarse, 1989).

In fact, subsequent experience cast doubt on whether this aim was achieved. For example, a case study of two large hospitals carried out in 1987 showed that their budgets increased by 15 to 17 per cent between 1983 and 1987 rather than being reduced by 7 per cent as official policy implied (Saltman and de Roo, 1989). The failure of policy seemed to result from cost-shifting strategies: namely, managers succeeded in undertaking new capital investments – for which addit-ional revenues were automatically approved – and by developing off-budget services which were beyond the regulators control.

This case study provides one example of the limited ability of official policy to address sources of macro and micro inefficiency within the health sector. A more general consideration of these inefficiencies is presented below.

Health sector failures

At the time of the publication of the reform proposals in 1987, the government argued that there were a number of health sector failings which needed to be addressed (Ministry of Welfare, Health and Cultural Affairs, 1988). These included: uncoordinated finance, few incentives for efficiency, unworkable government regulation and insurance market failures.

Different sources of health finance made it difficult to monitor, coordinate and control expenditure. Thus, for example, AWBZ had limited ability to control expenditure on nursing home care when it had no control or leverage over the decisions of individual doctors who placed people in nursing homes. In this way, separate budget responsibilities hampered attempts to increase efficiency through the substitution of different forms of care (Groenewegen, 1991).

Another problem was that the system contained few financial incentives for stimulating efficiency among providers, users and insurers. The fee-for-service system provided no incentive for hospital doctors to review their practice in order to eliminate unnecessary and inappropriate procedures. Quite the reverse: if anything, it encouraged oversupply. The formula through which hospital budgets were set made inpatient treatment more attractive than lower cost day surgery. Most patients had little reason to be concerned about the appropriateness and costs of their treatment, as their charges were close to being fully met by their insurers. Individual sickness funds received full reimbursement for their expenditures from the Central Sickness Fund and therefore had little incentive to improve their own efficiency or to seek to improve efficiency among the providers from whom they purchased services.

Government regulation had been used extensively in an effort to contain costs. This had included efforts to reduce the number of hospital beds, limits on hospital budgets and investment in new facilities, licensing of new technologies for reimbursement purposes, and the regulation of doctors' earnings through the negotiation of fee schedules. However, during the 1980s, concerns were expressed about the effectiveness of this approach (Rutten and Banta, 1988). Regulations were often unable to cope with the complexity of the health sector involving multiple groups, often with conflicting interests. Moreover, it often introduced perverse incentives, discouraging rather than encouraging efficiency, for example cost-increasing avoidance strategies and unintended distortions in resource allocation.

Insurance market failures in the Netherlands arose because of adverse risk selection and management inefficiency among the sickness funds. Adverse risk selection occurred because private insurers tended to cater for low risk individuals while sickness funds provided insurance for higher risk groups. A concern with equity meant that a complex system of compensation existed for transferring revenue from the private to the public sector. Management inefficiency among the sickness funds occurred because they operated as local monopolies with little need to compete for subscribers. One study indicated a variation of 69 per cent in the per capita expenses between the lowest and highest cost sickness funds (Kirkman-Liff and Van de Ven, 1989).

It was these sources of market failure that the health reforms set out to address.

The reform programme

The reform programme which began in 1989 was based upon three main principles. First, that there should be a basic health package available to all funded through social insurance. All existing financing should be channelled through a single system with sickness funds and private insurers competing for enrollees. Second, there should be a shift from government regulation to managed competition as a means of encouraging greater efficiency with appropriate financial incentives offered to users/consumers, insurers and providers of health care. Third, government regulation would still be used to ensure an acceptable quality of care and to meet various equity objectives such as local accessibility and solidarity between social groups.

Van de Ven (1990) pointed out that the links between the main groups of participants in the reform system could be viewed as three sets of bilateral relationships: namely, between consumers and insurers, insurers and providers, and providers and consumers (see Figure 8.1).

Consumers and insurers

The basic insurance package was designed to cover GP services, hospital charges and specialist fees, as well as nursing home care and certain forms of home care. To meet the costs associated with these services, all individuals would be required to pay an income-related premium into a central fund (an expanded version of AWBZ). Insurers – both sickness funds and private insurers – would then receive risk-adjusted, capitation payments from the central fund on behalf of those consumers who insured with them.

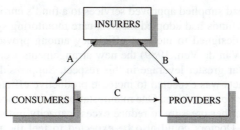

A: Insurers – Consumers (health care insurance)
B: Insurers – Providers (purchasing health care services)
C: Consumers – Providers (users of health care services)

Figure 8.1 **Relationships between consumers, insurers and providers**

The income-related premiums would be designed to cover 85 per cent of the costs of the basic package of care. The remaining 15 per cent would be raised in the form of fixed premiums paid directly by consumers to insurers. These payments would be unrelated to income and risk. Variations in fixed premium levels between insurers – based upon differences in management efficiency – would be expected to be one of the main sources of competition between insurers.

In addition to the basic insurance scheme, consumers would be free to take out supplementary private insurance to cover items not included in the basic package such as dental services for those over 18 years of age, physiotherapy and some medicines. Supplementary insurance would be financed by fixed premiums set by insurers.

Taken together, these insurance arrangements sought to combine efficiency, equity and choice. Income-related payments to the central fund were based upon ability to pay and would enable cross-subsidisation between individuals. Risk-adjusted capitation payments to insurers (together with open enrolment) were designed to reduce incentives for preferred risk selection. Competition between insurers for subscribers was expected to encourage them to operate more efficiently. Eventually the distinction between sickness funds and private health insurers was expected to disappear as they both competed for subscribers on equal terms. Finally, consumers would have choice between insurers and could purchase supplementary insurance if they wished to do so.

Insurers and providers

Under the new arrangements, insurers – both sickness funds and private insurers – would place service contracts with competing providers. Selective contracting would enable them to choose between providers on grounds of price and quality. This contrasts vividly with the pre-existing system where sickness funds were usually required to reimburse any provider that had supplied approved services to a fund's enrollee. While some sickness funds had adopted medical care monitoring systems and other devices designed to increase efficiency among providers (Kirkman-Liff and Van de Ven, 1989) the new arrangements were expected to give them far greater leverage in this respect. Supply-side competition for contracts was expected to increase productive efficiency in the use of resources by providers. One manifestation of this process was expected to be further pressure to reduce excess capacity in the supply of hospital beds. Doctors could also be expected to feel the pressure of competition. Fixed fees would no longer be guaranteed nor would new contracts with insurers be issued automatically.

Providers and consumers

Consumers would be able to choose the insurer and insurance scheme and, thereby, the provider from whom they wished to receive services. The quality of care offered by providers with whom particular insurers had contracts was expected to be an important consideration for consumers. If consumers were dissatisfied with the standard of care they received they would be able to change their insurer and/or provider. The ability of consumers to express their preferences in this way was expected to act as an important signal for the efficient allocation of health care resources. While the new emphasis upon managed competition was expected to shift the emphasis from regulated quality assurance onto consumer demand there would still be some cases where it would be necessary for the government to lay down minimum standards. For example, it was planned to use the Hospitals Facilities Act to provide for monitoring of large residential institutions. Beyond this, there was also some discussion of the need for government to support quality assurance through the development of accreditation schemes and other regulatory initiatives.

Analysis of the reform proposals

Van de Ven (1990) pointed out that the reform programme would have major consequences for insurers, providers and users of health care services.

Both sickness funds and private insurers would experience a marked change in their roles. Instead of fulfilling a primarily administrative function through the retrospective payment of claims, they would be expected to become cost-conscious purchasers of care. Their role would be far more active as a discriminating purchaser selecting among competing providers on grounds of cost and quality. Sickness funds would lose their regional monopolies and be required to compete with other insurers for enrollees. Similarly, private insurers would be faced with procompetition regulation such as open enrolment.

On the supply side, competition between providers for service contracts would also lead to changes in organisational behaviour. Hospitals would be required to respond to an external market environment in an entrepreneurial manner. Stronger internal management would be necessary to increase efficiency and price competitiveness. Doctors would also experience the pressures of competition as their incomes would be dependent upon hospitals' ability to attract contracts. These could no longer be expected to be obtained automatically.

Users of health care would also be confronted with cultural change. Far greater emphasis on choice – both as users of services and enrollees with insurance companies – would encourage active consumerism instead of a passive role as the recipient of services.

However, Van de Ven (1991) also noted that there were likely to be several problems associated with the transition from a centrally planned health care system to one based upon market principles. These related to consumers' lack of information, imperfect price signals and underdeveloped management skills.

In the Netherlands, as in most other countries, consumers rarely possess good information about health care services. This deficiency is particularly pronounced in relation to the quality of care. In part this reflects the inevitable complexity of quality measurement which manifests itself in multidimensional measures of structure, process and outcomes (Donabedian, 1982). The absence of well-informed consumers does, however, place limitations upon the efficient functioning of a market system. Consumer sovereignty is of questionable value when consumers do not have the information necessary to make wise decisions. Advocates of competition often argue that the process itself generates information and that rival providers and insurers can be expected to produce information in their quest to attract users and enrollees. It is, however, likely that independent accreditation agencies and other forms of quality assurance – involving additional, non-market mechanisms – will be necessary to supplement information supplied through the market.

The fact that prices within the Dutch health care system have been determined by negotiations between providers and insurers, and by government regulation, means that they have been poorly related to costs. As such, they could not be immediately relied upon to provide the right signals for achieving an efficient allocation of resources. Once again, supporters of the reforms believed that the competitive process would provide the necessary stimulus for the generation of better cost data. As the health care reforms in the UK and elsewhere have shown, however, this task requires heavy investment in information technology and the commitment of considerable quantities of other resources, both human and physical.

The need to develop better costing systems is closely related to the third factor that was expected to inhibit movement towards a market-based system, namely, the underdeveloped state of management skills in the health sector. Within the prereform systems, managers in hospitals and sickness funds had followed administrative procedures within largely bureaucratic structures. There had been little scope for managerial autonomy and discretion. Under the reform proposals, managers would be required to take responsibility for generating revenues and managing budgets. Moreover, human resource management – especially that involving clinicians who had traditionally enjoyed a large amount of professional autonomy – would become an important aspect of their work. Delivering the workloads negotiated through a contractual process would depend crucially upon clinicians and managers working to the same objectives. Inevitably a time lag could be expected to occur before the completion of the recruitment, education and training necessary to produce a cadre of managers with the skills required to carry out these tasks.

Another complicating factor surrounding the implementation of the reforms was the difficulty of determining a risk-adjusted, capitation formula for paying individual insurance funds from the central fund (Van Vliet and Van de Ven, 1992). Ideally, each insurer should receive a premium payment which reflects the risk category of the individual that insures with it. However, if these categories are set too broadly – such as on the basis of age and sex – the potential for preferred risk selection or 'cream skimming' is introduced. That is, insurers may select good risks (i.e. those people for whom the capitation payment is above their expected costs of care) and reject poor risks.

Cream skimming leads to a number of undesirable consequences (Van de Ven and Van Vliet, 1992). First, if the capitation formula does not adequately take account of health status, it is possible that people suffering from chronic disease or disability will experience reduced access to care. For example, insurers engaging in cream skimming would be likely to avoid contracting with providers who specialise in treatments for people suffering from cancer, heart disease or diabetes. Second, an imperfectly risk-adjusted capitation system could lead to efficient insurers being driven out of the market because investments in cream skimming might yield higher returns than investments aimed at genuine increases in efficiency. Third, cream skimming results in cost shifting. There is no net social gain as costs are shifted from one insurer to another. As such, resources devoted to cream-skimming activity are wasted when viewed from the perspective of the overall economy.

For these reasons, the effective prevention of cream skimming was seen by a number of Dutch health economists as a necessary condition for reaping the benefits of competitive health insurance within a regulated premium structure. Unfortunately, the government's approach was not seen by these economists as meeting this objective, primarily because it was based on a capitation formula in which age, sex and region were believed to explain a large proportion of the variance in health care expenditure. In fact the research evidence did not support this view.

Work carried out by Van Vliet and Van de Ven (1992) suggests that global variables such as age, sex and location can predict about one-fifth of the explainable variance in individuals' annual health care expenditure. However, if the previous year's expenditure incurred by individuals is added to the equation, the proportion of the explainable variance that can be predicted rises to three-fifths. If further indicators of health status and background characteristics are added, the proportion rises to three-quarters. These findings suggest that a variable reflecting prior expenditure should be added to the capitation formula in the short term. In the longer term, indicators of chronic health status should be added. Of course, these developments would involve substantial investments in data collection and administration.

Overall, therefore, technical problems associated with lack of information, imperfect price signals, underdeveloped management skills and the difficulty of devising a satisfactory capitation formula were all bound to slow the pace of implementation of the reforms. In addition, however, there were a range of broader economic, social and political factors which exerted an even more fundamental influence upon the pace of change. These factors are considered in the next section.

Progress (or lack of it) to date

The proposals for a market-oriented reform of the health sector, as set out in the Dekker Report, were widely discussed and debated during 1987. While there was general agreement about the need for reform, many individuals and organisations expressed reservations about the feasibility of implementing such radical change. Van de Ven and Rutten (1994) point out that the technical complexity of the reforms had been seriously underestimated. They argued that particularly complex problems were likely to arise in relation to the coordination of overlapping and sometimes inconsistent new and old regulations, in the definition of the benefit package to be covered by basic insurance, in the development and enforcement of an effective anticartel policy in health care and in fine-tuning policy to make sure that it was consistent with European Community regulations.

Moreover, many organisations suggested that the 'willingness to change' was not as widespread as the Dekker Committee implied (Bjorkman and Okma, 1995). In response to these concerns, the government organised a series of public hearings at which views and opinions could be expressed. Despite the expression of criticisms and/or fears on the part of patients' groups, workers and employers' representatives, and health professionals and providers, the main elements of the Dekker proposals were accepted by the Dutch parliament in 1988.

Two years later a new government comprising a Centre-Left coalition replaced the pro-reform Centre-Right coalition, but the main lines of the reforms continued to be accepted. However, it was noticeable that the 1990 proposals (referred to as the Simons Plan after the Secretary of State for Health, Hans Simons) employed a rather different vocabulary: reference to 'competition', 'markets' and 'incentives' was replaced by emphasis upon 'shared responsibility between parties', 'consumer choice' and 'decentralisation' (Van de Ven and Rutten, 1994).

According to the 1988 proposals, the reforms were due for completion by 1992. The 1990 proposals extended the implementation period for three years until 1995. However, it is now clear that even this proposal was over-optimistic. In 1993, Parliament set up an inquiry into the decision-making process in relation to health care reforms (the Willems Committee). In their report, published in 1994, the Committee concluded that there had been no clear political consensus for restructuring the health sector. Reforms had been hampered because different interest groups had been reluctant to look beyond their own narrow, parochial interests. This had led to some very vocal and effective opposition (Okma, 1995). As a result, neither of the fundamental proposals relating to basic insurance and regulated competition were realised.

A general election held in May 1994 resulted in a major loss for the two-party, Centre-Left coalition which was replaced by a three-party coalition comprising the Labour Party, the Liberal Democrats and the Liberal Conservatives. In September 1994 the new coalition presented its programme for the health sector. This departed from the route taken by their predecessors with greater emphasis being placed upon centralised regulation and planning. Thus a return to the pre-Dekker policy approach has been signalled.

Okma (1995) identifies six major interest groups that were particularly influential in opposing the implementation of the reforms. First, there were employers' associations that opposed the expansion of social insurance, fearing that this would lead to an increase in labour costs. Second, labour unions and consumer associations, while supporting the extension of health insurance, were concerned about the income distributional consequences of the flat rate premium payment component of the scheme. They feared that this would penalise low income groups and have an adverse effect upon social solidarity. Third, there was mixed support from hospitals and other providers about the introduction of supply-side competition. The proposal to end the mandatory contracting of hospitals by sick funds was seen as a particular threat to their financial base. Fourth, the medical professions also showed mixed support with some of their members opposed to the functional description of medical services. GPs were particularly vocal in their opposition to the redefinition of medical services and to proposals aimed at separating their funding sources from those of hospital consultants. Fifth, the sickness funds were divided. Although many of them were originally supportive of the proposal to create an integrated insurance scheme, reservations were expressed about the arrangements for nominal premiums, deductions and other copayments. There was also a concern on the part of the funds about the risks associated with some of the new insurance activities, particularly those involving long-term care. Finally, there was strong opposition to the proposals from the private insurance companies. They were concerned about the growth of bureaucracy, which they saw as being associated with the system of capitation payments. In the limit, they saw the proposals as heralding the end of the private insurance business and their future roles being relegated to one of managing a payment system within a publicly funded bureaucracy.

It would be wrong, however, to suggest that the ambitious proposals originally set out in the Dekker Plan have not resulted in any change. Several steps have been taken towards a more market-oriented system, especially in relation to the sickness funds (Van de Ven and Rutten, 1994).

For example, since 1993, sickness funds have received a partially risk-adjusted capitation payment from the central fund. Moreover, each subscriber is required to pay a flat rate premium (in addition to the income-related element) which is set by the individual fund. Since 1992, sickness funds have been able to sell policies on a nationwide basis, rather than being restricted to a single regional area. Entry to the sickness fund market has been made easier with several private insurance companies obtaining permission to establish new sickness fund organisations. Since 1994 sickness funds have been able to contract selectively with physicians and pharmacists. This represents a radical change from the situation that had previously been in force since 1941 and had placed a legal obligation on the funds to contract with each provider in their working area. Finally, since 1992, sickness fund members have been able to choose between different funds at least every two years. This has introduced an element of competition between sickness funds based upon their flat rate premium, quality, the providers with whom they contract, service responsiveness and reputation. Taken together, these changes mean that the sickness funds are in the process of moving from administrative bodies to competitive, risk-bearing enterprises.

Discussion

As was argued at the beginning of this chapter, the post-1987 period in the Netherlands offers a fascinating case study of the interplay between economic ideas and political realities within the health care sector. From the economist's perspective, the Dutch health care reforms represent a radical attempt to address the problems of aggregate cost containment and micro-inefficiency within the sector. They were produced at a time when several countries were looking towards competitive market solutions to these problems.

As Appleby has pointed out in Chapter 3, there is a well-established case for expecting markets to result in an efficient allocation of resources, as long as certain conditions are met. The Dutch reforms drew on these economic ideas and sought to reap the benefits of both demand-side and supply-side competition. On the demand side, there was to be competition from insurers for subscribers whereas on the supply side there was to be competition between providers for contracts from insurers. It was always recognised, however, that the health sector has certain special characteristics which prevent the simple adoption of market solutions. As a consequence a model of managed or regulated competition was proposed. The ideas of Enthoven (1986, 1988) were particularly influential in this respect, providing the outlines of a model of managed competition upon which the Dutch architects of reform were able to draw. In addition, however, the strong Dutch concerns about social solidarity led to the proposal for universal health insurance funded primarily on the basis of the ability to pay (i.e. income-related premiums).

Despite this clear focus on managed competition, as the account in the preceding section of this chapter has shown, it did not prove possible to implement the reforms in the way envisaged by the Dekker Committee. A number of technical factors and broader sociopolitical considerations have been identified as barriers to change. In the remainder of this section a closer look is taken at two of the reasons for this failure to convert the proposals into policy and practice. These are shifting attitudes towards competition policy and the barriers to change represented by the corporatist nature of Dutch society.

The Dekker reform proposals were conceived at a time when there was a worldwide move away from command and control systems towards market-based systems. There was a strong belief that a market-based, competitive environment provides the necessary incentive structure for greater efficiency. Throughout the 1980s this belief had provided the rationale for successive privatisation programmes around the world. This was the context in which Dutch and other policy makers turned their attention to the health care sector.

Health sectors in all OECD countries are noticeable for high levels of government intervention, involving different mixes of finance, direct ownership and regulation. As such, they proved to be a predictable (if somewhat late) target for those reformers who wished to introduce market-based reforms (Saltman and Von Otter, 1995).

Unlike other sectors of the economy, however, there was very little theoretical or empirical evidence to suggest that market solutions would result in greater efficiency within the health care sector. As Appleby (this volume) has pointed out, there is a well-established literature that documents the market failures that are endemic to the health sector. Moreover, as far as empirical evidence is concerned, the United States – which has relied upon market-based systems in health care to a far higher degree than any other OECD country – has been conspicuous for its failure to contain aggregate costs. Its performance in terms of micro-efficiency has also been far from impressive. Writing at the end of the 1980s, Zwanziger and Melnick (1988:305) summarised the US empirical evidence in the following terms:

The unanimity of the studies of hospital competition is striking; they have consistently found that hospitals operating in areas with greater competition tend to use more resources and to have higher costs. Despite the presence of methodological problems in all of these studies, they provide convincing evidence that competition will tend to increase costs in a market environment competing on non price bases.

Despite all of this evidence, however, the idea that markets and competition in health care can be expected to increase efficiency took hold. In seeking an explanation for this apparent contradiction, Moran has looked to broader questions of political economy (see Chapter 2). Whatever the strengths of this explanation, it is undoubtedly the case that the political dominance of the argument for market-based systems in health care has been tempered since the late 1980s. It has already been shown how, in the Netherlands, the language of the Simons Plan (1990) placed far less emphasis on market-based terminology than the earlier Dekker Report. (This mirrors a similar change over time in ministerial language in relation to the NHS reforms (Butler,1994).) Subsequently, this pull-back from a market approach was reinforced by the stance adopted by the three-party coalition elected in May 1994.

These developments signify a shifting attitude towards competition, indicating less willingness to accept it as a solution to the problems of the health sector. Paradoxically, this political shift seems to have taken place over the period when the emerging economic evidence is becoming slightly more favourable towards the case for managed competition, at least in the United States (Melnick and Zwanziger, 1995). Once again, this highlights the importance of the political determinants of change. In the Netherlands, health sector politics has reflected wider aspects of the Dutch political system.

In the previous section an account was provided of the major interest groups identified by Okma (1995) as posing barriers to health sector reform. These groups form part of a more general neocorporatist administrative structure within the Netherlands. Van der Grinten (1996) has summarised this structure in terms of a number of key characteristics. Three of these are of particular importance in analysing the slow progress of the Dekker reforms. First, within Dutch society there is an absence of a legitimised power centre for taking important decisions and implementing them. Second, there is a high degree of professional and organisational autonomy. Third, the administrative system is marked by a high degree of mutual dependency. This last feature means that, within the health care sector the government, providers of care and insurers are all dependent on one another to meet their own objectives. Their interaction has traditionally taken place in what is referred to as the 'social middle ground'.

The combined effect of these features is that it has been very difficult to implement radical change in the Netherlands. The recent history of the health sector provides a vivid example of the power of these constraints (Bjorkman and Okma, 1995).

However, Van der Grinten also argues that this system has come under pressure in recent years. He claims that there has been an erosion of the middle ground as individualism and decentralisation have assumed greater importance. Within the health sector, there has been a partial shift in the balance of power towards insurance companies and providers of care. These changes have loosened the constraints of neo-corporatism and introduced a greater element of uncertainty into the course of future policy. Quite how the mix of government regulation and market-based activity will evolve in the light of a weakened middle ground is difficult to predict.

References

Bjorkman, J.W. and Okma, G.H. (1995) *Restructuring Health Care Systems in the Netherlands: The Institutional Heritage of Dutch Health Policy Reforms*, (mimeo, unpublished).

Butler, J. (1994) 'Origins and early development', in R. Robinson and J. Le Grand (eds) *Evaluating the NHS Reforms*, London: King's Fund.

Dekker, W. (1987) 'Willingness to change' Bereidheid tot verandering; rapport van de commisserie structuur en Financiering Gezondheidszorg.

Donabedian, A. (1982) *Explorations in Quality Assessment and Monitoring. Volume II: The Criteria and Standards of Quality*, Ann Arbor, Michigan: Health Administration Press.

Enthoven, A. (1986) 'Managed competition in health care and the unfinished agenda', *Health Care Financing Review*, Annual Supplement, 105–110.

Enthoven, A. (1988) 'Managed competition: An agenda for action', *Health Affairs*, **73**:25–47.

Groenewegen, P.P. (1991) *Primary Health Care in the Netherlands: From Imperfect Planning to an Imperfect Market*? Paper for conference on 'Changing Roles of Government and the Market in Health Care Systems', Jerusalem.

Hoffmeyer, U.K. and McCarthy, T.R. (1994) *Financing Health Care*, Dordrecht, Netherlands: Kluwer Academic Publishers.

Kirkman-Liff, B.L. (1991) 'Health insurance values and implementation in the Netherlands and the Federal Republic of Germany', *Journal of the American Medical Association*, **265**(19): 2496–502.

Kirkman-Liff, B.L. and Maarse, H. (1992) 'Going Dutch', *Health Service Journal*, 24 September, 24–7.

Kirkman-Liff, B.L. and Van de Ven, W.P.M.M. (1989) 'Improving efficiency in the Dutch health care system: Current innovations and future options', *Health Policy*, **13**:35–53.

Maarse, J.A.M. (1989) 'Hospital budgeting in Holland: Aspects, trends and effects', *Health Policy*, **11**:257–76.

Melnick, G and Zwanziger J. (1995) 'State health care expenditures under competition and regulation, 1980 through 1991', *American Journal of Public Health*, **85**(10):1391–6.

Ministry of Welfare, Health and Cultural Affairs (1988) *Changing Health Care in the Netherlands*, Rijswijk: Ministry of Welfare, Health and Cultural Affairs.

Ministry of Welfare, Health and Cultural Affairs (1989) *Health Insurance in the Netherlands*, Rijswijk: Ministry of Welfare, Health and Cultural Affairs.

Okma, K.G.H. (1995) 'Restructuring health care in the Netherlands', in R. Williams (ed.) *International Developments in Health Care: A Review of Health Care Systems in the 1990s*, London: Royal College of Physicians of London.

Rutten, F. and Banta, H.D. (1988) 'Health care technologies in the Netherlands', *Journal of Technology Assessment in Health Care*, **4**: 229–38.

Saltman, R. and de Roo, A.A. (1989) 'Hospital policy in the Netherlands: The parameters of structural stalemate.' *Journal of Health Politics, Policy and Law*, **14**(4):773–95.

Saltman, R and Von Otter, C. (1995) *Implementing Planned Markets in Health Care*, Buckingham: Open University Press.

Schut, F.T., Greenberg, W. and Van de Ven, W.P.M.M. (1991) 'Anti-trust policy in the Dutch health care system and the relevance of E.E.C. competition policy and U.S. anti-trust practice', *Health Policy*, **17**: 257–84.

Towse, A. (ed.) (1995) *Financing Health Care in the UK: A Discussion of NERA's Prototype Model to Replace the NHS*, London: Office of Health Economics.

Van de Ven, W.P.M.M. (1990) 'From regulated cartel to regulated competition in the Dutch health care system', *European Economic Review*, **34**: 632–45.

Van de Ven, W.P.M.M. (1991) 'Perestrojka in the Dutch health care system', *European Economic Review*, **35**:430–40.

Van de Ven, W.P.M.M. and Van Vliet R.C.J.A. (1992) 'How can we prevent cream skimming in a competitive health insurance market?', in P. Zweifel and F.E. French (eds) *Health Economics Worldwide*, Dordrecht: Kluwer Academic Publishers.

Van de Ven, W.P.M.M. and Rutten, F. (1994) 'Managed competition in the Netherlands; lessons from five years of health care reform', *Australian Health Review*, **17**(3):9–27.

Van der Grinten, T.E.D. (1996) *Conditions for Health Care Reform. Changing the Policy System of Dutch Health Care*, Paper for Four Country Conference, 'Health Reform and Health Policy towards the Year 2000', Montebello, Quebec, Canada.

Van Vliet, R.C.J.A and Van de Ven, W.P.M.M. (1992) 'Towards a capitation formula for competing health insurers. An empirical analysis', *Social Science and Medicine* **34**(0):1035–48.

Zwanziger, J. and Melnick, G. (1988) 'The effects of hospital competition and the medicare PPS program on hospital cost behaviour in California', *Journal of Health Economics*, **7**(4):301–20.

Acknowledgements

I am grateful to Professor Ted Marmor and Ms Kieka Okma for comments and suggestions on an earlier draft of this chapter.

CHAPTER 9

Health reform in Sweden: the road beyond cost containment

RICHARD SALTMAN

Introduction

It has become something of a health policy truism to suggest that, if the 1980s was the decade of pursuing macro-efficiency at a system level, the 1990s has become the decade of pursuing micro-efficiency at the institutional level. Within this truism, however, individual countries have hewed out their own independent, sometimes idiosyncratic paths. Certainly, this has been true of developments within the Swedish health system. Sweden's overall policy trajectory bears considerable resemblance to that of other developed nations: indeed, it shares with the United Kingdom and the Netherlands the honour of being the first European country to embark on the micro-efficiency journey.[1] Yet the Swedish approach has provided an important counterpoint to the more dramatic – but in certain respects less successful – strategies selected in these other two countries. While the Netherlands sought with considerable trepidation to introduce competitive incentives on the funding side of its health system, Sweden has remained forthrightly attached to a tax-funded single-payer framework. While the United Kingdom has sought to professionalise (some would say corporatise) health sector management by insulating institutional governance from direct citizen influence, Sweden has further enhanced the directly democratic character of managerial decision making by decentralising practical authority to even lower levels of elected government. While both the United Kingdom and the Netherlands have, in the name of efficiency, further restricted the ability of patients to choose specialist level providers, Sweden has, in the names of equity and quality, broadened the ability of patients to choose both physician and institution within its publicly operated health system.

A constellation of political, economic and cultural influences have led Sweden down this broadly convergent yet intrinsically divergent health policy path (Saltman, forthcoming). These influences have often led Swedes, as embodied by their elected national, regional (county) and municipal representatives, to view the policy options for pursuing micro-efficiency rather differently from other counterpart OECD countries. The fundamental planned market questions have, of course, been similar across most publicly funded health systems (Saltman and von

Otter, 1995). They include, first, whether to adopt any form of competitive incentives at all within their health system; second, once competition is adopted as a strategy, whether to introduce it on the funding, production or allocation mechanism dimension of the health system (Saltman, 1994); third, if competition is to be adopted on the production side of the health system (as was the decision in the UK and Sweden), which actors should be incorporated into this new arrangement: general practitioners, hospital specialists, hospitals, nursing homes, home care services and so forth; fourth, what level and intensity of regulation, generally, and of standard setting, monitoring and evaluation specifically, is necessary to moderate opportunistic behaviour; and fifth, how to integrate pharmaceutical policy into the broader market/regulatory mix (Saltman and Kane, forthcoming).

The crucial question, in the Swedish case as elsewhere, concerns the long-term political and economic sustainability of these reform decisions, and the impact of micro-efficiency measures not only on institutional finances but also on the quality of care, and on equity and health gain. As the analysis below suggests, the Swedish path in pursuit of micro- as well as macro-efficiency has shown relatively good results thus far. Relatively good results, however, remain far from the requisite level that democratically accountable policy makers feel is sufficient. Further, the relative success of Swedish policy to date has now engendered a new set of policy dilemmas which, perhaps, Sweden will once again be among the first developed countries to confront.

Experience to date

Over the past 10 years, the Swedish health care system has changed dramatically on several important dimensions, yet changed hardly at all on other equally central parameters (see Box 9.1). How Swedish health policy analysts interpret the extent of change depends in considerable degree on their disciplinary preconceptions. Among public health advocates, who consider issues of equity and equality of health status to be the defining measurement of success, there is considerable worry that the pace of reform has been too rapid, and the consequences broadly negative (Diderichsen, 1995; Dahlgren, 1994). Swedish health economists, however, who consider issues of technical and dynamic efficiency to be the essential dimensions of measurement, contend that little real change has in fact occurred (Rehnberg, 1995; Anell, 1995).

Viewed conceptually, there has been substantial change in the allocation and production dimensions of the health system, but no change on the funding side, a pattern which parallels that observed in most OECD countries during this period (Saltman, 1994). On the production side, the delivery system is no longer frozen in a tightly planned web of producer-driven catchment areas with inconvenient access times. Considerable diversity across and within counties can now be found in the

---

Box 9.1: Before the reforms began

The Swedish health system in the mid-1980s was constructed upon a decentralised command-and-cantrol model of authority (Saltman, 1988). It was command-and-control in that nearly all planning and decision-making authority about the provision of hospital, primary and nursing home care in each of the 23 counties and three large municipalities was in the hands of a central publicly administered health and hospital care directorate. This directorate was account-able to an elected county council and was administered by a small number of elected members of the council, who became full-time county executives. It was decentralised in that each county owned and operated the hospitals and health centres within its boundaries, and contributed approximately 60 per cent of their running cost from a county council tax or personal income which it set itself. Moreover, under the terms of the 1982 Health Services Act, each county council had the right to decide how to organise its health services and the extent to which it wished to contract with private providers (typically nursing homes and private physicians). With the introduction of the Seven Crowns Reform in 1970, hospital physicians became county employees, as were most primary care physicians and nearly all auxiliary staff. Nearly all county council health personnel, including many administrators, were members of unions, which negotiated nationally about wages and working con-ditions with the Federation of County Councils. All county person-nel were paid on a fully salaried basis. Hospitals received a global budget, which was only indirectly related to the volume of services they provided. Patients were assigned by the county to health cen-tres and hospitals on a catchment area basis, and had no choice of either primary care or hospital physician. Social and home care ser-vices were the responsibility of the 254 municipal governments, and were linked to county-run health services through a set of co-ordination committees.

---

organisation and operation of providers. At the primary care level, some counties have privately managed group practices (Västmanland, for example), others allow for either private or public 'family doctors' rather than relying on the traditional structure of a publicly operated health centre. At the hospital level, institutions in a number of counties, while remaining publicly owned and operated, must now compete for patients and/or publicly placed contracts in order to meet their budgets. Patients in 1991 gained the formal ability to select care providers any-where in the country,[2] and in Western and Southern Sweden, cross-county provision has become quite normal as in each region several counties have begun the process of merging together (see below). Since formal contracts can only be indicative in such an organisational context, some subcounty districts have sought to develop contracts that offer higher quality and continuity of care as a way to entice patients to choose contracted providers (Malm, 1994, personal communication). Hospitals, in response to these pressures and incentives, have had no choice but to become less like bureaucratic agencies and more like public firms. Flexible management and more efficient use of personnel and resources have led to increases in productivity even as overall health expenditure as a percentage of GDP has fallen. In Stockholm County, productivity increased 11 per cent over a two year period in the early 1990s (Essinger, 1992, personal communication). In turn, increased productivity (stimulated in part by a special allocation from the national government) and patient choice combined to all but eliminate what had been up to two-year queues for elective procedures, especially for full hip replacement, coronary artery bypass grafts, and intra-ocular lens transplants. These improvements were achieved, moreover, while employment levels were being considerably reduced, as noted above.

One of the more indicative examples of the impact of market-style incentives on public providers is that of the 1982 Ädel Reform in the elderly care sector. Swedish hospitals at the beginning of the decade had as many as 25 per cent of their beds taken up by 'bed blockers', for example, elderly patients who were ready for discharge if the nursing home or home care services could accept them. The reform, based on an earlier experiment in North Jutland county in Denmark, involved two basic elements. Responsibility for operating the public nursing home, along with the requisite revenues, was transferred from the counties to the municipalities, so as to combine under one administrative roof all elderly residential services (old age homes, sheltered housing, and home care services as well as nursing homes). Municipalities were then required by law to accept 'finished' patients within five days of notification by the hospital. If they could not, the municipality would have to pay the full cost of continued inpatient care directly to the relevant county.

When the shift occurred in January 1992, the counties were quite convinced that they would receive substantial funds back from the municipalities, since they expected that there would still be a considerable number of elderly patients waiting in hospitals. Some counties went as far as to include these expected municipal payments in their prospective county budget. In the event, the municipalities were able to take responsibility for 85 per cent of these patients (Johansson, forthcoming). This reduction in patients, in turn, along with other micro-efficiency measures, left the hospital sector with an oversupply of inpatient beds which county administrators could then seek to close.

A second example of public sector flexibility in Sweden is the ongoing effort to reconfigure administrative responsibilities for the health sector at both regional (county) and municipal levels. At the regional level, as noted above, two groups of county councils have set in motion the process of merging into a new supra-county regional government. In the Göteborg area of Western Sweden, where five county councils have had an agreement allowing patients to obtain services anywhere in the five county region since 1985 (Västvenska Planeringsnämden, 1984), representatives will be elected in 1998 to a supra-county council. A similar process is under way in three counties in the Malmö region of Southern Sweden. One stimulus to this integration has been the advantages of scale in regional integration for the effective management of expensive hospital resources. A second influence has been the recognition, since Sweden joined the European Union in January 1995, that larger regional governments, capable of formulating regional development as well as health sector strategies, may become necessary if the power of national governments does in fact atrophy and a 'Europe of Regions' emerges.

The recentralisation of existing county councils into larger regional bodies has been accompanied by seemingly paradoxical efforts at continued decentralisation of county-run primary care activities to the municipal level. In addition to residential care for the elderly, in the 1992 Ädel reform, there is a new experiment in seven municipalities that pushes responsibility for primary health care down to the municipal level. Although an earlier effort, as part of the 'Free Municipality' experiment in the 1980s, did not lead to structural reform, there is some expectation that primary care will follow the same route as elderly services, an expectation that is heightened by the formation of supra-county regional governments. The old question as to whether the original county councils are too big to be local but too small to be regional appears to be re-emerging with a vengeance.

A third example of new-found flexibility in Sweden's publicly operated health system involves efforts in several counties to develop budgeting arrangements that strengthen the role of primary care vis-à-vis the hospital sector. The desire to create a primary-health-care-driven delivery system has been a part of the Swedish policy debate since 1948, when the notion was first raised in a report presented by Axel Höjar, director-general of the then National Board of Health (Serner, 1980). Elements of this approach were adopted in the 1974 Primary Health Care Act, which stipulated that increased emphasis was to be placed on the development of primary and preventative modes of care. In the early 1990s, counties like Kopperberg (since renamed Dalarna) and Stockholm adopted a series of budgetary mechanisms that had the effect of realigning the relationship between primary and hospital services. Utilising similar techniques, these counties gave most of the hospital budgets directly to subcounty primary care boards. These boards were responsible for providing primary health care services within their district, as well as contracting and paying for necessary hospital services. This reorganisation of the county budget transformed county hospitals into public firms that, instead of working from fixed global budgets, had to earn their revenues via patient choice of provider combined with public contracts from the subcounty boards. This had the effect of creating competition between the county's public hospitals for patient custom and revenue, and in turn putting pressure on hospital personnel to increase productivity and (to entice patients) enhance quality. A further intended effect is to encourage primary health providers to reduce unnecessary hospital referrals, as well as to expand the services they produce themselves, and thus to increase the cost effectiveness of the overall delivery system.

A fourth aspect of health policy in which reform has been introduced is pharmaceutical policy. In Sweden, as in other countries which have large pharmaceutical corporations, drug policy combines a concern to reduce the cost of domestically consumed pharmaceuticals with maintenance of an appropriate industrial policy to maintain employment levels and encourage pharmaceutical exports. Confronted with increasing pharmaceutical expenditures in the early 1990s, the national government adopted a reference pricing strategy that ties payment levels from public funds to the price of generic rather than brand name preparations (Ljungkvist *et al.*, forthcoming). In addition, after rejecting several proposals including one that would give primary care physicians an indicative budget for outpatient drugs, the Social Democratic government decided to separate patient cost sharing for drugs from that for outpatient physician office visits. Instead of having one combined ceiling for co-payments (which most recently had been 1,800 SEK a year, or approximately 250 USD), as of January 1997 there are now two separate co-payment ceilings, with a combined total not to exceed 2,200 SEK (approximately 325 USD) (Rothstein, 1996). While reference pricing has been shown to be effective in reducing overall expenditures without substantially affecting quality of care, increases in already high co-payments may affect equity (WHO, 1997), particularly given ongoing cutbacks in income transfer programmes.

In addition to organisational reforms, administrative reconfiguration and pharmaceutical policy, the pursuit of micro-efficiency in Swedish health policy has also included an enhanced national role for monitoring and evaluating both the quality and equity of health care reform. Concerns had been expressed about the increased diversity of service delivery arrangements across the counties, and in particular that decentralisation can lead not only to greater administrative flexibility but to fragmentation of services with different standards for different citizens depending upon where they live. Such fragmentation would break the legal commitment in the 1983 Health Services Act that entitled each citizen to receive 'care under the same conditions'. Responding to this concern, the National Board of Health and Welfare began an intensive programme of assessing health-related outcomes. The Board established six teams to examine outcome-related data, one for each region of the country, and conducts an intensive on-site assessment of each county once every three years. Subsequently, the Board has begun developing an intensified monitoring process that links outcomes to specific procedures, facilitating development of a set of best-practice protocols that counties are being encouraged to adopt (Örtendahl, personal communication, 12 September 1996).

Although the overall results of this period of health sector reform have largely been positive, this series of structural reforms has also generated its share of problems. Perhaps the most noticeable is the degree to which expenditure and cost containment issues have cast their shadow over the Swedish health policy landscape. This may be an unavoidable result of the serious 1991–93 recession combined with with continued growth in the demand for care. However, fiscal difficulties were undoubtedly exacerbated by a decision of the national government, for macro-economic reasons, to freeze county and municipal tax levels during the 1992–94 period. There is now some publicly stated concern that discussions of finance may be displacing efforts to resolve important service delivery questions.

Commentators have also paid attention to the degree to which political rather than care-related criteria have influenced decisions (Brommels, 1995). In the most notorious case of political factors overriding sound judgement, one Stockholm subcounty district let a contract for laboratory work to a private for-profit firm that lacked the necessary technical expertise and organisational infrastructure. Some six months later, a police raid was followed by disclosures that this firm had been mishandling blood samples and fabricating test results (Johansson, 1995; Läkaretidningen, 1996). The resulting scandal profoundly shook Swedish health policy makers, and served to underscore the importance of instituting strong public regulation over the small but (until then) growing numbers of private sector suppliers.

A third negative consequence of this reform period has been the inevitable consequences on employees of the success in increasing overall health sector productivity. Some 128,000 employees lost either full- or part-time jobs between 1990 and 1994, contributing to the rapid increase in overall unemployment in Sweden during this period. Since most of these workers received unemployment benefits, the overall financial benefit to the public sector of this reduction in force is considerably less than the savings in the health sector alone. Worried that overcapacity could lead county policy makers to close their facility, physicians and nurses are under pressure to reduce queues and to broaden service availability. Remaining employees have had to increase their workloads considerably, leading to concerns about employee overload and increased likelihood of professional 'burnout'.

Partly in response to these drawbacks of market-oriented health reform, and partly reflecting a renewed emphasis upon social solidarity as a result of the effects of the 1991–93 recession, health policy in the most recent 1994–96 period has shifted away from competition-based approaches. Signalled by the 1994 electoral victory of the Social Democratic Party, not only at the national level but also in 25 of 26 county councils, the key phrases in health policy circles have reverted to 'cooperation' and 'coordination'. This philosophical return has not reversed the ongoing processes of administrative reorganisation and cross-sector budgetary incentives already in place. Rather, it indicates a turning back to basics, a focus on the core cultural values that have motivated Swedish health service arrangements for several generations. It also demonstrates the residual belief of many county-level politicians that reimposition of tighter command-and-control forms of administration is the only feasible response to the combination of a shortfall in financial resources and increasing demands for service. In some counties, this has gone so far as to produce statements from county administrations that they may seek to eliminate patient choice of providers. It seems extremely unlikely, however, that such a step would actually be taken. There is continued strong interest on the part of Swedish citizens in having new and better sources of information upon which to guide their choice of provider (Anell and Rosén, 1996). The democratic structure of governance in the Swedish health system suggests that it will not be politically possible for administrators to re-impose tight catchment-area controls on the citizenry even were they to desire to do so. Some county politicians, moreover, continue to recognise the fiscal and managerial benefits that have been achieved within a controlled, public competition environment, particularly for acute hospitals, and are unlikely to contemplate a move backward to the inefficient 'frozen' administrative structure of the 1980s.

In this context, it should be noted that the private sector of the Swedish health care system has remained small throughout the reform period. Although several private insurers and providers had high expectations at the beginning of the competition-oriented reform period in the early 1990s (Mosten, 1990, personal communication), their forecasts have turned out to be largely incorrect. On the funding side, the number of new private health insurance policies was estimated in 1992 at 45,000 (Rosenthal, 1992). Most commentators believe this figure has substantially gone down as a result of the severe 1991–93 recession. However, the impact of current financial constraints as well as the return of queues for some elective procedures could, if not countered, result in the number of private policies starting to grow again.

With regard to hospitals, as noted above, there is a new diversity in the delivery arrangements in the public sector, including several public hospitals that have been dramatically reduced in size and then placed under private management (for example, Sabbatsberg in Stockholm). Efforts by conservative politicians in some counties to place large clinical facilities under private management have, however, mostly failed. The most telling case in point was Sankt Görans Hospital in Stockholm, where negotiations with an international hospital management company foundered on demands by the company that it receive a guaranteed revenue stream from the county – something no publicly operated hospital could receive given the county's large budget deficit – and when it became apparent that the management company's expected rate of profit would result in higher overall costs to the county for running the hospital. Despite this lack of penetration of the public sector at the level of clinical services, there has been over the past several years an appreciable increase in private contracting for support services such as cleaning and catering.

With regard to privately owned hospitals, the two small pre-existing private facilities – in Stockholm and Göteborg – remain open; however, several newer start-up efforts ended in bankruptcy. It is interesting to note that new private hospitals have recently suffered a similar fate in Finland and Denmark, raising an important question for those who believe that privately operated facilities are by definition more efficiently operated than hospitals in the public delivery system.

With regard to private outpatient physician specialist services, there has been noticeable growth, largely in the cities. Beyond efforts by county councils such as Västmanlands to establish privately operated county health centres, efforts to set up private polyclinics in more sparsely populated areas have frequently failed. In rural Dalarna County, for example, two separate efforts to establish a private polyclinic in Falun, to take advantage of the new contracting role of the subcounty primary care boards, ended in bankruptcy. City Akuten, a chain of walk-in clinics for primary care services founded in 1983, continues to do well, in part because they have been able to maintain county payment from public funds for the private services provided.

Emerging issues

It is no small irony that as cost-related issues have risen to the top of the health policy agenda, Sweden's overall health expenditures, calculated as a percentage of GDP, have fallen. Among OECD countries, Sweden's performance regarding aggregate health expenditures has been noticeably the best. While expenditures have been upward in most developed countries in the first half of the 1990s (OECD, 1996), those of Sweden have dropped appreciably. From 9.4 per cent of GDP in 1980, the figure fell to 8.6 per cent in 1990 and to 7.4 per cent in 1995 (Berleen, personal communication, 15 October 1996). This figure is now well below the overall Western European average, which for 1994 was 8.0 per cent of GDP (WHO, 1997). Even after allowances for the effects of the 1992 Ädel reform, which resulted in approximately a 0.9 per cent reduction in the GDP health figure due to the transfer of funding for nursing homes to the municipal social budget (following the Danish pattern), the overall change during this 15-year period has been a reduction of 1.1 per cent. The fact that this reduction was achieved, despite the broad economic effects on county budgets of the 1991–93 recession, further demonstrates the extraordinary character of the achievement.

This reduction in the overall rate of health expenditure has, in turn, raised a variety of new health policy issues that can be expected to grow in importance over the remainder of the decade. In essence, these issues pose the basic question, 'After cost containment succeeds, then what?' (von Otter, 1997, personal communication). The policy dilemmas can be summarised in three related categories:

• the sustainability of low expenditures;
• potential options for raising new health-sector revenue;
• alternative arrangements to absorb unemployed workers in home and social care jobs.

Each is discussed in turn.

The sustainability of low expenditures

The difficulties presented by Sweden's march down to 7.4 per cent of GDP have begun to make themselves visible. While there are other concurrent pressures that share in the responsibility, the overall picture is of a system under strain. One indicator is that during 1996, there have been increasing reports at the county level of a return of patient queues for certain elective procedures. In Stockholm County, which struggled in 1995 with a one billion SEK (150 million USD) deficit, the closing of a third acute care facility (Lowenströmska) has resulted in some of the remaining hospitals becoming overcrowded (Berleen, personal communication, 15 October 1996). There has been intensified discussion about the impact on quality of care if current budget levels are maintained. Projections by the Federation of County Councils indicate that many counties will be operating with substantial deficits by the year 2000 (Haglund, personal communication, 25 March 1996), and some counties face continued budget reductions in the next several years (Brogren, personal communication, 3 July 1995).

Looking to the long-term consequences of tight revenues, a Swedish commission on priority setting was established in 1992. While its final report has been praised for its emphasis on equity, in practice the report identifies only a few medically marginal procedures that might be candidates for elimination from public funding (SOU, 1995:5). The Swedish priorities report, however, like its counterparts in the Netherlands and elsewhere, failed to address the real world consequences of a shift from implicit (e.g. physician-determined) to explicit (e.g. politically-determined) rationing of publicly funded health services. Once public payment is discontinued, financially better-off citizens will most likely purchase either supplementary insurance or needed care directly from their personal resources, while the financially less well-off will have no similar alternative. Thus, despite stated concerns regarding equity, the introduction of explicit rationing would inevitably translate into real reductions in service only for poorer citizens, and would thus increase this group's already disproportionate burden of ill health.

More broadly, the central question is how tightly public budgets and services can be squeezed before middle-class Swedes will rebel, either by making political demands for higher levels of public expenditure, or by redirecting part of their personal disposable income toward the purchase of private insurance or services.

Potential options for raising new revenue

The dilemmas created by potential options to raise new revenues for the Swedish health sector parallel the issues raised by similar questions in other European countries. In the face of intensifying globalisation of the world economy, with increased competitive pressures on both the price and quality of exports, a relatively small country like Sweden that has a relatively high proportion of exports feels itself particularly vulnerable. Simultaneously, the intensification of regional integration, in the form of the single market in Europe, has the same effect of heightening competitive pressures. Economists argue that, to respond effectively to both pressures, Sweden (like other countries) must increase the proportion of its GDP invested in private industry so as to enhance quality and productivity. In turn, public sector expenditures like those on health would have to be reduced as a proportion of total national spending. This competitive market argument dovetails with the fiscal policy requirements laid down in the 1992 Maastricht Treaty of the European Union for the approaching 1999 European monetary union. Annual budget deficits and aggregate national debt must both be reduced, to 3 per cent and 60 per cent of GDP respectively. The current Swedish Prime Minister, Göran Persson, has made major strides in meeting both these targets since he took office in March 1996. Indeed, successful budget tightening in combination with an improved economy led Persson to announce in January 1997 that a 10 billion SEK (1.3 billion USD) surplus existed, which would be devoted to easing the worst funding problems in the health and education sectors (*Financial Times*, 23 January 1997). However, there is little room for dramatically increased public spending on health in upcoming budgets. Thus, Sweden's political adherence to the European Union in 1995 has severely restricted the possibility of finding new public funds for support of the health sector without further drastic cuts in transfer payments or other welfare state services.

Conversely, most Swedish health policy makers, and especially the Social Democratic politicians who currently lead all but one county council, see new private funds not as a potential solution but as a danger to be avoided. Although co-payments have increased marginally in Sweden (as in the case of pharmaceuticals), the overall percentage of health expenditures composed of patient fees has risen only from 2 per cent of expenditure in 1987 to 3 per cent in 1993 (Spri, 1996). Also, as noted earlier, private commercial health insurance is not a likely source of new health funding (barring substantial further reductions in public sector expenditures), a situation welcomed by the majority of Swedes who equate increased private insurance with a breakdown in solidarity and equality.

Of course, there is a natural tension between the level of public funding and the likelihood that private individual mechanisms will take root. Experience in the Netherlands suggests that the publicly funded system must provide a similar service standard to that available from private commercial insurance if the solidarity of the public system is not to be decreased by middle-class citizens deciding to, in effect, buy their way out through the purchase of private commercial insurance (de Roo, 1995).

With both increased tax revenues, as well as private individual funding either not feasible or unavailable, new options will necessarily revolve around some hybrid of collective yet nonpublic resources. One option may lie in adapting the long history of cooperative movements in Sweden, which still include a number of agricultural producer cooperatives as well as the large consumer federation (Kooperativ Förbundet) which operates nationwide grocery and superstore chains. A new cooperative mechanism could perhaps be designed at municipal level that could raise additional funds for health sector use that would then spread the benefits from these funds to all residents. Another option would be to tie a new insurance structure to union membership (von Otter, 1997, personal communication). While the design of such a supplemental system of collective yet nonstate revenues is not at this point clear, the need for new resources to maintain existing standards of quality of care and to forestall socially divisive rationing is becoming increasingly apparent. If the response to this funding shortage is not to fragment into individual solutions based on personal income, this or some other type of community-based arrangement will be needed.

Alternative arrangements for unemployed workers

The third policy dilemma is perhaps the most painful. Sweden now has its highest rate of both real (8 per cent) and buffered (6 per cent in job training programmes) unemployment since the 1930s. If the Swedish welfare state model is to sustain itself, this level of unemployment is both socially and financially unsustainable. Consequently, a large number of new jobs must somehow be created. In current economic circumstances in a developed European country like Sweden, the necessary growth will have to be in the service sector. With the continued ageing of the population 18 per cent of Swedes are over 65 years old, compared with 12 per cent in USA and 11.7 per cent in Japan), the strong present and inevitably increasing demand for health-related human services such as social and home care services, points to an obvious fit that would be both socially as well as economically beneficial: pay these unemployed individuals to work in the social care sector. Under present budgetary structures, however, this is difficult to do. Swedish policy analysts have begun to call for the creative redirection of existing unemployment insurance funds to create long-term social and home care jobs (von Otter, personal communication 12 June 1995; Rothstein, 1996), and some health sector labour unions like SKAF have now developed their own model for this type of programme (van Otter, personal communication, 1997). Such schemes may become complicated if there is resistance from other labour unions to what they perceive as less skilled and, perhaps, lower paid competition to their own workers. Moreover, such ideas could founder again – as they did in the early 1980s with a proposal for a national service approach to providing social and home care (Secretariat for Future Studies, 1984) – on the fear that such new workers would be uninterested in the work and would provide poor quality services. A new source of health-related funding is likely to be necessary, therefore, if the new service sector jobs to be created are not to be only in franchise food and other commercial sectors of the economy, but are also to draw on this obvious resource to help resolve a pressing human services problem.

Conclusion

As the above analysis suggests, the three policy dilemmas that the Swedish health system confronts are closely interrelated. The potential unsustainability of the current low level of health expenditures; persistent demand for new care producers, particularly in social and home care services; the availability of a pool of unemployed workers; and the necessity of developing a new collective nonpublic but nonprivate funding source, all reflect different aspects of the same central issue. If the Swedish health care system is to sustain its present level and quality of service, there will need to be substantial readjustments to health sector resources. Reform efforts from the early 1990s demonstrate not only the degree of improvement which could be made, but, in the mid-1990s, the subsequent shift back toward a more middle path suggests that many, if not most, organisational micro-efficiencies may now have been achieved. While there will always be additional measures to be taken, they are likely to produce diminishing returns, and thus to be incapable of resolving the central dilemma the system now confronts.

Even with the post-1994 shift back to a broad policy focus on co-operation and coordination, there has nonetheless already been substantial change in the Swedish health system's overall organisational pattern. Patient choice, introduced in 1991, is likely to grow rather than diminish in influence. Hospitals, health centres and other provider institutions will continue to be funded in ways that are more tightly linked to productivity, with an increasing number assuming the de facto status (if not the title) of public firm. It is also likely that recent experiments in decentralising hospital budgets to primary care boards will continue and, most likely, broaden.

Some critics of the Swedish system's reforms have described them as a 'boomerang', arguing that they have failed and that the health system has now returned to its original position (Dahlgren, personal communication, 13 November 1996). It may well be that the more applicable metaphor is Hegel's dialectic. If the health system in the early 1980s was the thesis, and the more market-influenced reforms of the early 1990s the antithesis, then one could consider the emerging arrangement to be the synthesis. Whether and/or how stable this synthesis will be, however, inevitably depends on the answers which national policy makers develop in the three linked dilemmas that the health system now confronts.

Notes

1. The United States, of course, pursued institutional level micro-efficiencies throughout the 1980s, however it did so in an incoherent manner that undermined rather than reinforced macro-efficiency.
2. The counties, acting through the Federation of County Councils, accepted a resolution at their annual congress stating that patients should have freedom of choice of provider. Some counties have not publicised this right, and others, faced with fiscal stringency, have tried to discourage cross-county care. Additional restrictions were introduced in 1995 and 1996 in some counties.

References

Anell, A. (1995) 'Implementing planned markets in health services: The Swedish case', in R. B. Saltman and C. von Otter (eds) *Implementing Planned Markets in Health Care: Balancing Social and Economic Responsibility*, Buckingham: Open University Press.

Anell, A. and Rosén, P. (1996) *Valfrihet och Jamlikhet i Varden*, Stockholm: SNS Forlag.

Brommels, M. (1995) 'Contracting and political boards in planned markets', in R.B. Saltman and C. von Otter (eds) *Implementing Planned Markets in Health Care*, Buckingham: Open University Press.

Dahlgren, G. (1994) *Framtidens sjukvardsmarknader: vinnare och forlorare*, Stockholm: Natur och Kulture.

de Roo, A (1995) 'Contracting and solidarity: Market oriented changes in Dutch health insurance schemes', in R.B. Saltman and C. von Otter (eds) *Implementing Planned Markets In Health Care*, Buckingham: Open University Press.

Diderichsen, F. (1995) 'Market reforms in health care and sustainability of the welfare state: Lessons from Sweden', *Health Policy*, **32**:141–53.

Johansson, A.(1995) *Dagens Nyheter*, 5 March, p. 6.

Johansson, L. (forthcoming) 'Cost and utilization of pharmaceuticals in

Sweden', in R. B. Saltman and N. M. Kane (eds) *Comparative Experience in Pharmaceutical and Home Care Policy*, Supplement, *Health Policy*.

Läkaretidningen (1996) 'Flera hundra förfalskade provsvar lämnade laboratorie företaget', *Läkaretidningen*, **93**:532

Ljungkvist, M.-O. *et al.* (forthcoming) 'Cost and utilisation of pharmaceuticals in Sweden', in R. B. Saltman and N. M. Kane (eds) *Comparative Experience in Pharmaceutical and Home Care Policy*, Supplement, *Health Policy*.

OECD (1996) *Health Data Base*, Paris: OECD.

Rehnberg, C (1995) 'The Swedish experience with internal markets', in M. Jerôme-Forget, J. White and J. M. Weiner (eds) *Health Care Reform through Internal Markets: Experience and Proposals*, Washington D.C.: Brookings Institution.

Rosenthal, M. (1992) 'Growth of private medicine in Sweden: The new diversity and the new challenge', *Health Policy*, **21**:155–66.

Rothstein, B. (1996) 'Debatt', *Dagens Nyheter*, 15 October, p. 4.

Saltman, R. B. (1994) 'A conceptual overview of health care reform', *European Journal of Public Health*, **4**:287-93.

Saltman, R. B. (1998) 'Sweden', in R. B. Saltman (ed.) *International Handbook of Health Care Systems*, Westport, Connecticut: Greenwood Press.

Saltman, R. B. (forthcoming) 'Convergence vs. social embeddedness: Debating the future direction of health care systems', *European Journal of Public Health*.

Saltman, R. B. and Kane, N. M. (eds) (forthcoming) *Comparative Experience in Pharmaceutical and Home Care Policy,* Supplement *Health Policy*.

Saltman, R. B. and Figueras, J. (1997) *European Health Care Reform: Analysis of Current Strategies*, Copenhagen: WHO.

Saltman, R. B. and von Otter, C. (eds) (1995) *Implementing Planned Markets in Health Care: Balancing Social and Economic Responsibility*, Buckingham: Open University Press.

Secretariat for Future Studies (1984) *Time to Care*, Oxford: Pergamon Press.

Serner, U. (1980) 'Swedish health legislation: Milestones in re-organisation since 1945', in A. J. Heidenheimer and N. J. Elvander, (eds) *The Making of the Swedish Health Care System*, New York: St Martins Press.

SOU (1995) *Priorities in Health Care: Ethics, Economy, Implementation*, SOU: Stockholm.

Spri (1996) *Health Care in Sweden: The Facts*, Stockholm: Spri.

Västvenska Planeringsnämden (1984) *Regionsjukvardsavtal med dartill knutna avtal for vastra sjukvardsregionen*, Goteborg: Vastvenska Planeringsnamden.

von Otter, C. (1996) 'Den Planerade Marknadeu', in *Om Nye Styformer i Halsö- och Sjukvården*, Stockholm: National Board of Health and Welfare.

WHO (1997) *European Health Care Reform: Analysis of Current Strategies*, edited and written by R.B. Saltman and J. Figueras, Copenhagen: WHO.

Acknowledgements

Valuable comments on an earlier draft of this chapter were received from Casten von Otter and Wendy Ranade.

CHAPTER 10

The German Model: the state and the market in health care reform

RICHARD FREEMAN

Introduction

In the comparative study of the health sector, a number of factors make the German example more than usually interesting. First, its size: Germany's is the largest system in Europe, covering 80 million people. Second, it was the first European country to develop state regulation of the provision of health services: it was 'the pioneer in national health care' (Leichter, 1979). Third, it has served as a policy model, both in the period of welfare state foundation and since. Indeed, it is the prime example of what has been described as the 'public contract' pattern of the finance and provision of health care, that model on which other European systems are currently seen to be converging (OECD, 1992; Hurst and Poullier, 1992).[1] The German example has also been at the centre of recent reform discussion in the USA (cf Navarro, 1991; Albritton, 1993).

To what extent is the provision of health care in Germany ordered by market mechanisms? To what extent, and why, has the number and/or significance of those market mechanisms been increased by recent reforms? This chapter sets out by providing a schematic account of the 'German model'.[2] It describes core arrangements for health finance through the compulsory insurance system, for the provision of medical services by hospitals and by doctors in local practice, and for the supply of medical goods (principally pharmaceuticals). It discusses the mechanisms by which the system operates and is regulated, that is, in political terms, the way it works. It describes pressures for reform and subsequent legislation. It comments on the political process by which reform has been achieved, and concludes with an assessment of recent changes.

The German model

The lynchpin of health care in Germany is the statutory system of health insurance (the *Gesetzliche Krankenversicherung*, GKV) by which it is financed. Over 99 per cent of the population is insured against health risks, 88 per cent in the GKV. Its stipulated benefits cover treatment (prevention and screening; physician and hospital services; contraception, abortion and sterilisation) as well as income supplements (sick pay, maternity benefits). Only high earners are allowed to rely on private insurance arrangements, which are usually nonprofit schemes. Seventy-five per cent of the population, those earning up to a fixed ceiling, are compulsorily insured in the GKV while a smaller number (12–13 per cent) are voluntary members choosing to be insured in the GKV rather than privately (OECD, 1992).

The GKV is composed of a large number of independent sickness funds, which are of two kinds: regular funds (RVO or *Reichsversicherungsordnungskassen*), mandated by social insurance legislation, and substitute funds (*Ersatzkassen*). Regular funds include local or district sickness funds, company or factory funds and others catering for specific occupational groups such as miners, farmers and seamen. These cover 60 per cent of the population, including both blue and white collar workers. Substitute funds, which are former mutual aid schemes and usually have a nationwide organisation, cater for a further 28 per cent of the population, mainly white collar employees. There are approximately 1,300 funds in all, 1,100 in the western Lander and 200 in the new Lander in the East (Schulenburg, 1994).[3] There is a limited element of competition within and between different kinds of funds for voluntary members: different schemes tend to compete by offering higher optional benefits as well as by reducing contributions (Pfaff, 1990).

Insurance contributions or premiums are financed in equal shares by employers and employees and are paid on earnings up to a fixed ceiling. Contribution rates are fixed by individual funds in order to cover the collective costs of their members: in 1992, contributions averaged 12.9 per cent of gross income (OECD, 1992). The payments made by GKV funds to providers account for 60 per cent of health care finance; federal, state and local government investment and payments to providers for a further 21 per cent; user charges for 11 per cent and private insurance (including both patient reimbursement and payments to providers) for 7 per cent. Total health spending in 1990 amounted to 8.7 per cent GDP (Table 10.1).

The provision of health care in Germany is clearly separated between hospital and ambulatory services. Hospitals provide very little outpatient care. Public hospitals are owned by regional and local authorities (51 per cent beds) and by nonprofit organisations (35 per cent beds). Some are run as businesses (14 per cent beds) and are owned mostly by groups of medical professionals (OECD, 1992). The sector as a whole is characterised by a large number of hospitals with low average bed capacity, and the ratio of beds to population is high. Hospital operating costs are met by sickness fund payments, and capital costs by regional and local governments. Hospitals receive a fixed fee for each day a bed is filled, which makes for some incentive to oversupply.

German physicians are either hospital employees or work independently in local, private practice. There are more specialists (60 per cent) in local practice than general practitioners (40 per cent). Individ-

Table 10.1 **Total health spending and statutory health insurance (GKV) spending, per cent GDP, Federal Republic of Germany, 1970–1990**

	Total health spending	GKV spending
1970	6.4	3.7
1975	8.3	5.9
1980	8.0	6.1
1985	8.5	6.2
1986	8.6	6.2
1987	8.7	6.2
1988	8.9	6.4
1989	8.3	5.8
1990	8.7	5.8

Source: Reiners, 1993.

ual patients are free to choose (and change) their doctor, though they must stay with one doctor during any one accounting period (three months). There is some competition between doctors for patients, which has been intensified by a marked increase in the numbers of doctors entering medical practice (Moran, 1990). The instruments of this competition – higher rates of prescription and hospital referral, and greater investment in and use of medical technology – represent a significant cost pressure (Pfaff, 1990).

Membership of their respective regional Association of Sickness Fund Physicians permits individual doctors to treat sickness fund patients. The associations must accept qualified doctors, who therefore hold both the right and an effective obligation to membership. The associations are required to plan the supply of medical services to meet demand, such that the care to which sickness fund members are entitled is in fact provided. The associations are legally responsible to the funds, who are in turn responsible to their members.

Doctors' earnings are derived from a fee-for-service system, while being ultimately constrained by global budgeting. Medical procedures are allocated a point value on a nationally agreed rating scale. The monetary value of points is fixed by negotiation at regional state level, and varies between states accordingly. If the collective fees charged by physicians in any one state exceed the total amount contracted between the funds and the physicians' association, the association reduces the point value.[4]

How does the system work? As described here, the German health care state is divisible into a number of highly regulated subsectors or interlocking fields in which specialised health care goods are produced, delivered and paid for. Like any system, it is made up of a number of component parts; like any system, too, what defines it is not simply the specific character of parts but the relationships between them. These can be described as corporatist and federalist in turn.

The production and distribution of health and medical services in

Germany is ordered not by price but by negotiation.[5] Payments to providers are set in the course of negotiations with payers; they are not the result of marketplace activity. Negotiations take place at regional level between groups of sickness funds and physicians' associations, within what has been described as a 'highly formalised' relationship (Hurst, 1991). Other negotiations take place at local level between funds and hospitals, reflecting what amounts to a bilateral monopoly (Hurst, 1991; OECD, 1992).[6] This is a kind of institutionalised collective bargaining (Döhler, 1991) characteristic of corporatism.

A more general 'concert' of negotiations is achieved in different ways (Henke, 1986; Döhler, 1991; Schulenburg, 1992). Principal among these is a process of concerted action established under the terms of the 1977 Cost Containment Act (Henke, 1986). The Concerted Action committee constitutes a national arena in which policy development is discussed by representatives of the major players involved in the finance, delivery and regulation of health care, including pharmaceutical companies as well as doctors' organisations, hospitals, sickness funds and governments.

Government power as such is diffused across federal, state and local tiers. The federal government is reponsible for health policy in general and for health legislation and jurisdiction. Professional and pharmaceutical regulation, hospital finance, medical research and contagious diseases legislation were formerly the responsibility of a department of health at the Federal Ministry of Youth, Family Affairs, Women and Health; these were taken over by a separate Ministry of Health formed in 1990, which also took responsibility for sickness insurance regulation, previously part of the social insurance remit of the Ministry of Labour and Social Affairs. Regional state governments approve federal legislation (in the parliamentary second chamber, the Bundesrat); supervise negotiations between physicians' associations and sickness funds; take responsibility for hospital planning and investment as well as for managing state-owned hospitals; and regulate medical education, which brings indirect control of the supply of doctors through manipulating the enrolment of medical students. In some states, public (environmental) health is devolved to the municipalities. A standing Conference of Ministers of Health of the regional states holds a further informal coordinating function.

In this way, the system is regulated through what are for Germany characteristically federalist and corporatist processes (Busse and Schwartz, 1995). It is essentially ruled by law: the power to mandate procedural changes in the system lies with federal legislature. Responsibility for its operation, for administration and implementation, lies with the funds and with doctors, according to a principle of corporatist self-government (*Selbstverwaltung*).[7] The fragmented nature of health corporatism, however – a fragmentation by design which results partly from German federalism but also from the 'segmentation' (*Gliederung*) of the statutory insurance system into different kinds of fund including the separation of finance from delivery and of ambulatory from hospital care – makes for a large number of actors in health politics, in turn making corporatism seem much more like pluralism. Concerted Action, for example, is a corporatist institution which works in a pluralist way. As a result, the German health sector may best be described as an 'arena of struggle over the distribution of burdens and benefits' (Moran, 1990: p 2). The aim of the rest of this chapter is to show how, in the process of current reform, it remains an 'arena of struggle' rather than a market.

Reform pressures

The system has a number of acknowledged performance weaknesses. These include a certain lack of equity both in terms of finance between members of different kinds of sickness fund and in terms of service provision between different geographical areas (below), but primary among them is the problem of cost (Moran, 1992; OECD, 1992; Schulenburg, 1992). What is seen to be excessive cost inflation is attributed to a lack of cost consciousness among both providers and users (Henke, 1990) and to the oversupply of hospital beds and physician services. Longstanding concern with cost is evidenced by legislation passed in 1977, 1982 and 1983 and supplemented by hospital reform during 1982–86 (Hurst, 1991) (Box 10.1).

Price stability was slowly established during the 1980s (Table 10.1). An 'income-oriented expenditure policy' was expressed in a commitment to a stable health insurance contribution rate (*Beitragssatzstabilität*) (Reiners, 1993). Legislation in 1988 mandated that sickness fund expenditure should not increase faster than wages. In 1991, however, spending by statutory sickness funds grew more than twice as fast as wages (Stillfried and Arnold, 1993) and control of contribution rates was legislated for explicitly at the end of 1992.[8]

The relationship between cost and reform is an ambivalent one. The legislative programme of cost containment is recognised as a success (Schneider, 1991; Schulenburg, 1994). German health spending reflects its size and wealth and, in relative terms, is consistent with that of other European countries. Yet it remains an incipient cause for concern. In part, this reflects Germans' awareness of the costs of health care: though money may matter little to providers and users, sickness insurance contributions are effectively a health tax, the burden of which is visible on every wage-slip. But unions, employers and the federal government share an interest in restricting nonwage labour costs, of which health and social insurance contributions are a growing part. Limits to increases in health insurance contributions are political as well as economic, and are increasingly self-evident. In this context, the focus of continuing concern in the health sector becomes its internal cost efficiency rather than its overall cost as such.

This question of finance is related to questions of equity. Relatively

Box 10.1   Health reform in the Federal Republic of Germany 1975–90

1977   *Health Insurance Cost Containment Act*
- introduces principle of income-oriented expenditure policy;
- creates Concerted Action forum for interested parties in health sector;
- re-introduces lump-sum prospective budgets for payments from sickness funds to doctors' associations;
- strengthens medical audit (utilisation review of physicians);
- introduces negative list for drugs and raises pharmaceutical co-payments;
- requires nursing care in some circumstances to be provided at home rather than in hospital;
- requires family members with income above certain level to pay separate insurance premium;
- introduces risk-sharing scheme across funds in respect of pensioner members.

1981–82   *Supplementary Cost Containment Acts*
- introduces patient co-payments on medical aids and appliancs and transport to hospital, extending them for drugs, physiotherapy and glasses.

1982   *Hospital Cost Containment Act*
- extends domain of Concerted Action to hospital care;
- requires that per diem rates for inpatient stays be negotiated between hospitals and sickness funds;
- involves sickness funds in regional states' hospital planning.

1983–84   *Amended Budget Acts*
- introduces charges for hospital inpatient care;
- extends co-payments for drugs;
- requires that old age and unemployment insurance contributions be paid from sickness benefit.

1985   *Hospital Financing Act*
- shifts mixed federal and regional state financing of hospital building to regional states.

1986   *Federal Hospital Payment Regulation*
- introduces prospective global budgets for hospital operating costs, to be negotiated between hospitals and sickness funds, while allowing for special daily rates for expensive kinds of care.

Box 10.1 continued

1986   *Need Planning Act*
- restricts registration of new doctors in some specialisms in some areas where overprovision already more than 50 per cent.

1988   *Health Care Reform Act (Gesundheitsreformgesetz, GRG)*
- mandates that sickness fund expenditure should not increase faster than wages;
- introduces reference prices for nonpatent drugs and other medical goods;
- provides for closer monitoring of physician prescribing and extension of quality assurance in both hospital and ambulatory care;
- reforms the independent medical advisory service to sickness funds;
- obliges doctors to consider the cost effectiveness of referrals against published hospital price lists;
- allows sickness funds to end contracts with uneconomic hospitals;
- extends co-payments for hospital stays and patient transport in particular;
- sets income ceiling for compulsory contributions by waged workers and raises pensioner contributions;
- extends provision of preventive health care as insurance benefit;
- provides financial support for carers of long-term sick;
- announces future, more fundamental reform of organisational structure of sickness funds.

Sources: Schneider, 1991; OECD, 1992; Schulenburg, 1992.

low earners paying in to local funds with higher burdens of risk among their memberships inevitably pay higher rates of sickness insurance than others; in 1993, contributions ranged from 10.8 per cent to 16.4 per cent of gross wages (Schulenburg, 1994). Following unification, the higher levels of morbidity and mortality, combined with (and related to) lower incomes among the population of the former East Germany, have made the issue of the differential risk burden between funds more acute.

A different order of problem has less to do with performance as such than with responding to weakness. The organisational fragmentation (above) which inhibits policy making and implementation itself constitutes a policy problem. In a cumulative process begun in the postwar period (Schulenburg, 1992), law-making in health in Germany has expressed a continuing 'search for control' on the part of government. Health politics is essentially *Ordnungspolitik*: it is the function of the state to structure and maintain a particular economic order, in this case the social market (Maneval and Neubauer, 1982). And in order to fulfil this function, the state must be able to assert some regulatory authority. In this context, reform of the system is always likely to have as much to do with the identity of parts and the relationships between them as with their immediate function.

Reform

Major legislative reform of the health sector in Germany was introduced in 1988 and 1992. In 1988, a Health Care Reform Act introduced reference prices for drugs; required closer monitoring of the quality and quantity of physician services, as well as of numbers of doctors; increased freedom of negotiation for sickness funds in relation to hospitals and medical referrals to hospital; made some adjustment to the list of benefits provided under compulsory health insurance and extended cost-sharing (Box 10.1). In 1992, the Structural Reform of Health Care Act restricted the growth of health spending to the growth of sickness fund revenues; relaxed the former strict demarcation of hospital and ambulatory care in the interest of improved coordination and reduced duplication of services; fixed doctor-to-population ratios; required that any overspend of newly fixed drug budgets be repaid by doctors' associations and the pharmaceutical industry; introduced risk pooling between sickness funds to improve equity; introduced freedom of movement for workers between different kinds of fund; laid the basis for the prospective amalgamation of funds and brought some marginal increase in cost sharing (Abel-Smith and Mossialos, 1994) (see Box 10.2).

The 1992 reform was the first to change the structure of the German health system since its foundation in 1883. It impinged directly on the institutional organisation of health insurance, and the ways in which doctors are paid. Whatever ministers' intentions – and Blüm in 1988 had clearly set out to achieve fundamental change (Webber, 1989) – previous reform had been effectively 'structure-neutral' (Bandelow, 1994). Its historic significance lies in large part in its erosion of the class stratification of health insurance, without which the structure and development of the system can scarcely be understood.

The keynote of the GSG was the extension of specific forms of competition to the finance of health care. Following the reform of health care in 1988, patients were obliged to pay the difference between fixed prices and actual prices for prescription drugs, a move which was intended to introduce price competition among pharmaceutical producers (Schulenburg, 1992). In 1992, they were to be free to choose between insurers while the funds, for their part, were to be compensated for the differential burdens of their memberships by a national risk-adjustment scheme. As Health Minister Seehofer claimed, 'Risk adjustment and

Box 10.2   The structural reform of health care, 1992

Gesundheitsstrukturgesetz (GSG)

Physician services
- service fees fixed at 1991 levels, and tied to increase in fund revenues until 1995;
- replacement of fee-for-service by mixture of capitation and 'service complex' payments;
- hospitals allowed to provide outpatient care, physicians in local practice to perform operations outside hospitals;
- increase proportion of doctors in primary care, increasing their fee levels, limitations placed on numbers of doctors by establishing doctor-to-patient ratios.

Hospital finance
- introduction of payment by diagnosis rather than bed-day by 1996;
- intention that hospital capital as well as current expenditure be financed by sick funds rather than regional states.

Pharmaceuticals
- regional drug budgets fixed, with first DM280M overspend to be reimbursed by doctors' associations and second DM280M by pharmaceutical industry;
- positive list pharmaceuticals to be introduced in January 1996;
- reference pricing extended, while prices of nonreference priced drugs reduced and frozen;
- indicative drug budgets for individual practitioners.

Sickness funds
- risk-adjustment subsidies between funds, beginning 1994.

Health care users
- free movement between funds for insured members;
- increase patient co-payments.

Sources: Abel-Smith and Mossialos, 1994; Schulenburg, 1994.

consumer choice make for a new competitive order which improves the conditions for economic efficiency and contributes to downward pressure on contribution rates' (Seehofer, 1993: 102).[9]

Since January 1996, blue collar workers and the retired and unemployed have been allowed to choose (and move) between local and other funds, a choice previously allowed only to white collar workers. Funds themselves must accept any applicant (Abel-Smith and Mossialos, 1994). The risk-adjustment scheme compensates funds for their relative burdens of risk indicated by the demographic profile of their members according to age, sex, income and numbers of co-insured dependants. It therefore equalises those factors intentionally kept beyond funds' control. Some funds become net contributors under the scheme, some net beneficiaries.

The reform has been vilified on two counts, which may be mutually contradictory. First, it is said to undermine solidarity among fund members, in that the activation of consumer interest makes sickness insurance seem an individual rather than collective proposition.[10] Second, it is seen to standardise national health insurance, in a way which inhibits rather than promotes competition. Sickness funds' freedom to negotiate the range of services they offer to members and the prices they pay to providers has become increasingly restricted by federal legislation (Schulenburg, 1994; Busse and Schwartz, 1995). The calculation of insurance premiums as well as benefit packages, service pricing and administrative organisation have become more regulated and uniform (Schulenburg, 1994). Meanwhile, the competition between GKV and private insurers is limited by the progressive reduction – a concomitant of the universalisation of public health care – of that proportion of the population not compulsorily insured in the GKV.

> Although the reformers claim to be generating equal conditions for competition between the funds before introducing unlimited choice between statutory health insurers, they have effectively standardised all activities of the funds. This opens up the prospect of a single national sickness fund in the near future.
>
> (Stillfried and Arnold, 1993: 1017)

The 1992 Act facilitated the amalgamation of local sickness funds and it seems that numbers of local sick funds might be reduced from 270 to 20–30 (Abel-Smith and Mossialos, 1994). Competition, which in theory produces variety, is predicated on uniformity.

In a similar way, a new system of payment for inpatient care and a new freedom to make profit is expected to stimulate the development of a private sector in hospital care (Schulenburg, 1994). Budgets which were formerly fixed for each hospital individually, in negotiation with sickness funds, have been replaced for 1996 by a system which combines case fees, procedure fees and departmental day rates. Case and procedure fees are fixed centrally, by the Federal Ministry of Health, leaving only departmental day rates subject to local negotiation (Busse and Schwartz, 1995).

In more general terms, the introduction of competition to a highly regulated market may have perverse effects and may fail to increase efficiency. Where the scope for competitive advantage has been taken away, competition leads to inefficiency, for example by artificially or needlessly inflating marketing budgets. With this in mind, the federal government froze the administrative costs of sickness funds for the period 1993–95 (Schulenburg, 1994).

Reform process

Legislative activity over a 20-year period constitutes what may be described as a routinisation of health reform in Germany, which may be understood in different and perhaps complementary ways.

First, repeated reform attempts seem to testify to their repeated relative failure. At the end of the 1980s, with Norbert Blüm outmanoeuvred by the health political lobby, it was difficult not to see the post-1975 period as one of reform blockade (Rosewitz and Webber, 1990; Webber, 1988, 1989). The essential organisational logic of corporatism is conservative: its most influential players tend to be committed to obstructing reform and to maintaining an existing order, as were the substitute funds in 1988 (Bandelow, 1994).

Second, and at the same time, such lengthy reform processes almost inevitably offer some evidence of gradual, incremental change. There are many instances of ideas being introduced by government at one stage, only to be realised much later. The Federal Hospital Payment Regulation of 1986, for example, encouraged hospitals to begin keeping statistics on the diagnosis, speciality, age and length of stay of patients (OECD, 1992). Cost-per-case pricing, however, which is predicated on the availablity of such information, was legislated for in 1992 to be introduced in 1996. Similarly, and more generally, the 1992 Act clearly signalled further cost containment legislation for 1996 and 2000.

Third, the perpetual prospect of reform may lead health interests to make the kind of calculation which game theory might predict. The effect of the announcement and discussion of legislation to come sometimes seems to be greater than that of new legislation itself (Schulenburg, 1994). It is the uncertainty of major players in the health system, all the time wanting to avoid restrictive legislation, which inhibits their profit-maximising behaviour. In turn, legislation is followed by a process of adaptation to new rules under which each player seeks to gain maximum advantage. It is well recognised that Concerted Action, in so far as it works at all, works only through moral pressure and the incentive of participants to avoid more intrusive cost containment legislation (OECD, 1992).

Fourth, the Structural Reform of Health Care in 1992 generated changes of a degree which require interpretation of a different, more immediate kind. While Blum's reform had foundered on the health political lobby (Webber, 1989), what is distinctive about 1992 was the exclusion of sectional interests and the prominence of parties (Bandelow, 1994). A new health minister, Horst Seehofer, was appointed early in 1992 to a coalition cabinet committed to health reform. Its initial proposal said nothing about organisational change, to which the liberal FDP, a minor party but the keystone of the governing coalition, was resistant. That proposal was duly rejected by the SPD and the regional states, the majority of which were now SPD governed, and a Social Democrat counter proposal argued for the organisational reform of the sickness funds. The government offered a cooperative agreement, aware that a risk-adjustment scheme and wider access to different funds would be conditions of Social Democrat participation. A cross-party meeting took place in October 1992 in Lahnstein, and legislation was approved by the Bundesrat as soon as December. The reform arena belonged to the parties, not the sectional interests of Concerted Action (Bandelow, 1994).[11]

Fifth, and in sum, reform redirects attention to the role of the state in health policy. The German health sector is regulated by a peculiar combination of hierarchies and networks (Thompson *et al.*, 1991), in which the state appears as the 'architect of associational order' (Döhler, 1991, 1994).

Reform, the model and the market

While the advocates of market solutions to putative health sector problems typically originate among health economists or the neo-liberal political Right, what is interesting here is that, in Germany, neither quarter championed the market. Neoconservatives were never able to dominate the process of policy formulation in the governing CDU (Döhler, 1991), while the most influential school in health economics is led by a theory of 'nonmarket economics' (Döhler, 1994). Nor was there any private sector pressure for expansion (Döhler, 1991). In Germany, 'Cost-containment policy has been primarily price containment policy' (Schneider, 1991: 96): this containment has been achieved less by deregulation than by strengthening capacities for regulation. While reform has introduced some elements of competition to the German health sector, these in no way add to any existing commodification of health goods. Simply, they cannot be said to constitute a 'market'.[12]

Successive reforms have incorporated an element of reprivatisation of the costs of health care. The prosolidarity financing of social insurance is being hollowed out by increasing copayment obligations (Hinrichs, 1995). But reprivatisation of this kind remains conceptually and programmatically distinct from marketisation. Perhaps even more significantly, in imposing strict material and procedural provisions, the Structural Reform of Health Care in 1992 represented 'the state's recovery of strategic capacities and autonomy against the priority of self-government in the health care sector'(Hinrichs, 1995:671). The political conditions of the introduction of competition merely reflect what has become almost a truism: that the free market is predicated on the strong state (Gamble, 1988). But this prompts a further question: to what extent can a market predicated on a strong, interventionist state be described as a market, let alone as 'free'?

As this chapter has tried to show, any market elements of the finance and delivery of health care in Germany are firmly embedded in other modes of coordination represented by hierarchies and networks (Sayer,

1995; Thompson *et al.*, 1991). To some extent, this is quite usual: 'the state is a normal feature of real markets, as a precondition of their existence. Markets depend on the state for regulation, protection of property rights, and the currency' (Sayer, 1995: 87). Most markets, however, are only regulated on the supply side, while buyers retain the freedom to move between them. What is not normal is that negotiation which takes place between a single (group) buyer and a single (group) seller and which forms the basis of the German health system. If this can be described as a market, it is one which is not merely regulated, but rigged (Sayer, 1995).

Notes

1. Characteristic of this model are 'sickness funds, financed by compulsory, income-related contributions, which contract directly with independent providers for services supplied free of charge to patients' (Hurst and Poullier, 1992: 179; OECD 1992: 137).
2. What follows here is a highly schematic account, written for the purpose of this volume. For fuller introductions, see Moran (1992, 1994), OECD (1992), Schneider (1991), Schulenburg (1992, 1994). For detailed treatment of competitive and market elements, see Pfaff (1990).
3. What is remarkable about the unification process is that it now warrants little more than a footnote in descriptive accounts of health care in Germany. As in other areas, health political unification has amounted to a colonisation of the former East Germany by the organisations, practices and interests dominant in the West.
4. David Wilsford describes this mechanism as a 'global volume envelope' (Wilsford, 1994: 280, note 8).
5. The system has established 'comprehensive insurance coverage and freedom of choice but no free market on prices. Prices for medical services are set by negotiated fee schedules, per diem rates or other statutory pricing rules' (Schulenburg, 1992: 716).
6. Deborah Stone refers to a 'monopoly franchise' (Stone, 1991: 403).
7. The wider application of these principles in German social policy is discussed in Freeman and Clasen (1994).
8. One of the formal aims of the Structural Reform of Health Care was the '*Sicherung der finanziellen Grundlagen der GKV und Beitragssatzstabilität*'.
9. 'Mit dem Risikostrukturausgleich und der Kassenwahlfreiheit wird eine neue Wettbewerbsordnung geschaffen, die die Bedingungen für Wirtschaftlichkeit verbessert und den Wettbewerb über günstige Beitragssätze fördert' (Seehofer, 1993: 102).

10. See Hinrichs (1995) for extensive discussion of the threat to the 'moral infrastructure' of the health care state.
11. Medical interests were similarly excluded from the reform of the NHS in the UK 1989–91.
12. In that restricted sense, recent changes owe as much to Darwin as to Adam Smith.

References

Abel-Smith, B. and Mossialos, E. (1994) 'Cost containment and health care reform: A study of the European Union', *Health Policy*, **28**: 89–132.

Albritton, F. P. (1993) *Health Care Insurance Reform in the United States. A market Approach with Application from the Federal Republic of Germany*, Lanham, Maryland: University Press of America.

Bandelow, N. (1994) 'Ist Politik wieder autonom? Das Beispiel Gesundheitsreform', *Gegenwartskunde*, **4**:445–56.

Busse, R. and Schwartz, F. W. (1995) 'Germany: Hard choices ahead', *European Health Reform*, **2**:6–7.

Döhler, M. (1991) 'Policy networks, opportunity structures and neo-Conservative reform strategies in health policy', in B. Marin and R. Mayntz (eds) *Policy Networks: Empirical Evidence and Theoretical Considerations*, Frankfurt: Campus.

Döhler, M. (1994) 'The state as architect of political order: Policy dynamics in German health care', paper presented at ECPR workshop The State and the Health Care System, ECPR Joint Sessions of Workshops, Madrid, 17–22 April.

Freeman, R. and Clasen, J. (1994) 'The German social state: An introduction', in J. Clasen and R. Freeman (eds) *Social Policy in Germany*, Hemel Hempstead: Harvester Wheatsheaf.

Gamble, A. (1988) *The Free Economy and the Strong State: The Politics of Thatcherism*, Basingstoke: Macmillan.

Henke, K.-D. (1986) 'A "concerted" approach to health care financing in the Federal Republic of Germany', *Health Policy*, **6**: 341–51.

Henke, K.-D. (1990) 'Respondent: Federal Republic of Germany', in OECD (1990) *Health Care Systems in Transition. The Search for Efficiency*, Paris: OECD.

Hinrichs, K. (1995) 'The impact of German health insurance reforms on redistribution and the culture of solidarity', *Journal of Health Politics, Policy and Law*, **20** (3): 653–87.

Hurst, J. (1991) 'Reform of health care in Germany', *Health Care Financing Review*, **12** (3): 73–86.

Hurst, J. and Poullier, J.-P. (1992) 'Paths to health reform', *OECD Observer*, **179**: 4–7.

Leichter, H. M. (1979) *A Comparative Approach to Policy Analysis. Health Care Policy in Four Nations*, Cambridge: Cambridge University Press.

Maneval, H. and Neubauer, G. (1982) 'Ordnungspolitik und Gesundheitssektor in der Sozialen Marktwirtschaft', *Medizin, Mensch, Gesellschaft*, **7**: 172–8.

Moran, M. (1990) *Distributional Struggles in the German Health Care System: Cost Containment and the Doctor Glut*, University of Manchester: EPRU Working Paper 2/90.

Moran, M. (1992) 'Between the lines: Germany's problems of success', *Health Service Journal*, 23 April: 20–23.

Moran, M. (1994) *'Health care policy'*, in J. Clasen and R. Freeman (eds) *Social Policy in Germany*, Hemel Hempstead: Harvester Wheatsheaf.

Navarro, V. (1991) 'The West German health care system: A critique', *International Journal of Health Services*, **21**(3): 565–71.

OECD (1992) *Reform of Health Care: A Comparative Analysis of Seven OECD Countries*, Paris: OECD.

Pfaff, M. (1990) 'Market elements and competition in the health care system of the Federal Republic of Germany', in A. F. Casparie, H. E. G. M. Hermans and J. H. P. Paelinck, (eds) *Competitive Health Care in Europe. Future Prospects*, Aldershot: Dartmouth.

Reiners, H. (1993) 'Das Gesundheitsstrukturgesetz – ein "Hauch von Sozialgeschichte"? Werkstattbericht Über eine gesundheitspolitische Weichenstellung', WZB papers P93–210, Berlin: Wissenschaftszentrum Berlin für Sozialforschung.

Rosewitz, B. and Webber, D. (1990) *Reformversuche und Reformblockaden im deutschen Gesundheitswesen*, Frankfurt: Campus.

Sayer, A. (1995) *Radical Political Economy : A Critique*, Oxford: Blackwell.

Schneider, M. (1991) 'Health care cost containment in the Federal Republic of Germany', *Health Care Financing Review*, **12**(3): 87–101.

Schulenburg, J.-M. Graf v d (1992) 'Germany: Solidarity at a price', *Journal of Health Politics, Policy and Law*, **17**(4): 715-38.

Schulenburg, J.-M. Graf v d (1994) 'Forming and reforming the market for third-party purchasing of health care: A German perspective', *Social Science and Medicine*, **39**(10): 1473–81.

Seehofer, H. (1993) 'Neue Wettbewerbsordnung in der GKV erfordert größere Flexibilität', interview, *Die Ortskrankenkasse* (DOK), **3**: 101–3.

Stillfried, D. von and Arnold, M. (1993) 'What's happening to health care in Germany?', *British Medical Journal*, **306**(6884): 17–18.

Stone, D. (1991) 'German reunification: East meets West in the doctor's office', *Journal of Health Politics, Policy and Law*, **16**(2): 401–12.

Thompson, G., Frances, J., Levacic, R. and Mitchell, J. (eds) (1991) *Markets, Hierarchies and Networks. The Coordination of Social Life*, London: Sage/Open University Press.

Webber, D. (1988) 'Krankheit, Geld und Politik: zur Geschichte der Gesundheitsreformen in Deutschland', *Leviathan*, **16**(2): 156–203.

Webber, D. (1989) 'Zur Geschichte der Gesundheitsreformen in Deutschland – II Norbert Blüms Gesundheitsreformen und die Lobby', *Leviathan*, **17**(2): 262–300.

Wilsford, D. (1994) 'Path dependency, or why history makes it difficult but not impossible to reform health care systems in a big way', *Journal of Public Policy*, **14**(3): 285–309.

Acknowledgements

I am grateful to Viola Burau and Russell Keat for research material and to Karl Hinrichs for comments supplied for an earlier draft of this chapter. Remaining errors of fact and interpretation are my own.

CHAPTER 11

Conclusions

WENDY RANADE

In this final chapter I try to answer the questions posed in the beginning of the book, in the light of the evidence and theorising presented earlier. First of all, were there common pressures or triggers for reform and if, as Moran suggests, these lay in changes in the global economy, how were these experienced by the different states and mediated through the ideological perceptions of national policy elites? Secondly, what explains the emergence of the new market orthodoxy as a response to these pressures in the absence of any evidence as to its feasibility or effectiveness? Thirdly, what kind of market incentives were used and with what objectives in mind? Finally, and most important of all, what were the outcomes both intentional and unintentional, and hence the lessons reformers might draw from the market experiment?

The pressures for reform

Moran's chapter shows how, at a macro level, pressures for cost containment in health care are intimately linked to changes in the global economic order, the intensification of competition and organisation of production. The growing interdependence of national economies, exposed to global processes of production and competition, limits the freedom of individual states to pursue fiscal and monetary policies to support high welfare spending, and as capital flows to the most productive and profitable states so governments have to discipline the environment to avoid capital flight and attract direct foreign investment. Since health care is a major component of the budgets of all mature welfare states, it is hardly surprising that it received such sustained attention from policy makers.

The precise nature and timing of these pressures, however, depended on each state's position in the international economy. The severity of economic crisis and decline experienced by New Zealand and the UK partially explains their early status as radical pioneers in health sector reform. The strengthening of the European Union can itself be seen as a counter-response to the intensification of global competition and power of transnational capital. The attempt to deepen political and economic interdependence of the member states through the Single European Market in 1992 and (for some members) meet the Maastricht criteria for entry into the European Monetary Union by 1999 helps to explain the wider context in which cost containment in health spending was pursued by states like The Netherlands and Germany (although the unexpectedly high costs associated with re-unification is also important in the German case). In addition it conditioned the response of Sweden, with its high marginal tax rates and levels of public spending, entering the EU in 1995.

In the United States, the perception that high health care costs borne by employers was hindering the competitiveness of American industry in its struggles with Japanese rivals was part of the reason for the growing national consensus that *something* must be done about health sector reform which, as Marmor's chapter shows, provided the Clinton administration with what turned out to be the mirage of an opportunity. In the Canadian case, health care reform was intricately bound up with Canada's continuing constitutional crisis but here too economic pressures began to unwind the system of 'fiscal federalism' which had guaranteed the essential features of the health care system across the country.

The workings of democratic politics and interparty competition for votes may, however, moderate the radicalism suggested by economic pressures, as seems to have been the case in New Zealand and the UK and, more recently, in some of the Canadian provinces. European research suggests that majorities of two-thirds or more of EU citizens believe their government should maintain social protection even if that means higher taxes, with support for expanding welfare strongest in the lowest spending countries – including the UK – and lowest in the highest spending countries like the Netherlands (Taylor-Gooby, 1996). At the same time, in mature capitalist democracies more assertive and sophisticated 'citizen-consumers' have become dissatisfied with the rigidities and inefficiencies of traditional public service bureaucracies, demanding more choice and higher quality services (Ridley, 1996).

The converse of more educated and assertive users of health care is a decline in the cultural and professional authority of doctors, though this can also be linked to a number of other factors: challenges from other health care professions, particularly nursing (Witz, 1991); the rise of alternative medicine and self-help as a response to the perceived failings of orthodox medicine (Saks, 1991); growing scepticism among policy elites about the 'scientific' basis of medical decision making on effectiveness and efficiency grounds; and the rise of the 'corporate rationalisers' – managers and health economists – as a response. In some countries, notably the UK but also New Zealand and the USA, the authority of doctors has also suffered from neoliberal ideological attacks on the power and motives of producer groups, and it is in these countries that market-oriented doctrines of public management have found their most zealous proponents. Taken together, these forces have upset the established balance of interests within the health sector, and the normative pattern of relationships which regulated it.

But if these factors help to explain the context in which health sector

reform became more pressing and opened up opportunities for new reform directions, they do not fully explain why market-based approaches
became fashionable, in spite of evidence of their equity and efficiency
failings. There are different levels of explanation for this policy paradox. Moran explains it at the level of political economy, stressing the
structural embeddedness of health care in capitalist democracies as concentrations of economic and political power in their own right, and the
dilemmas and contradictions facing policy makers trying to reconcile
competing strategic interests, in particular, the need to support technological innovation in the medical goods industries to foster success in
export markets with the need to curb demand for the products of this innovation at home. Market ideologies appeared to address these dilemmas
by promising policy makers new ways of rationing demand when traditional control systems (based on the authority of doctors) were eroding;
protecting and creating further opportunities for private capital in providing
goods and services[1] or like 'managed competition' promised the efficiency gains of markets without their equity disadvantages.

Economic and political dilemmas are, of course, refracted through
ideological lenses. The global context at the end of the 1980s was the
collapse of communist states in Eastern and Central Europe, the seem-
ing final victory of capitalism (Fukuyama, 1992) and the triumphalism
of its promoters. In the Anglophone countries it would be surprising if
prolonged New Right attacks on the values and institutions of the welfare state had not undermined solidarity and confidence in the efficacy
of state action to meet social need. (In the USA of course this was never
pronounced in the first place.) What is more surprising is the extent to
which public opinion in the UK, Canada and New Zealand has with-
stood these attacks, yet as Moran and other authors point out, support
for public health care systems is increasingly conditional on performance, with sections of a more prosperous and expanding middle class
readier to turn to the market to buy a high quality or quantity of service.
In Germany, the Netherlands and Sweden, the values of solidarity are
still strong but similar strains are still evident. Indeed one of the key dilemmas posed by the Swedish case is how to reconcile cost containment
and efficiency improvement in the public health sector with middle-
class aspirations for choice and high quality services in the longer term.

Appleby (Chapter 3) argues that the UK's success in privatising or
de-regulating large sections of state industry, policies subsequently
rolled out throughout the world, made it an influential policy leader and
role model in public sector reform, and provided the leap of faith
necessary to think the unthinkable: if competition worked in other
fields, why not in health care too? The case studies provide plenty of
evidence of policy learning between countries, and considerable traffic
in ideas and personnel between them. International bodies like the
OECD have been influential both in defining the problems to be addressed and the solutions to be adopted, first stressing the problems of
ageing populations (1988) then high levels of unemployment and the

need to sustain economic competitiveness (1994a). The OECD consistently argued for retrenchment and restructuring of social welfare systems and the need to devolve some responsibilities to the private sector (Taylor-Gooby, 1997). At the same time it was influential in disseminating information on health reform strategies to a wide audience at reg-ular intervals (OECD, 1987, 1992, 1994b). Marmor and Maynard (1994) also stress the role of international management consultancy companies in the dissemination of market prescriptions for public sector reform.

But, as Klein (1995: 98) points out, receptivity to foreign ideas is not neutral but depends on how far they reinforce or contradict current ideological values and prejudices in the importing countries. Hence the importance of the Reagan–Thatcher ideological closeness, and the traffic in ideas to Britain largely from America, which were later influential in Sweden, New Zealand and the Netherlands (Marmor and Plowden, 1991). The influence on public sector reform, including health care, of American-trained neoliberal officials in the New Zealand Treasury is also noted by Campbell (1995). Yet as Klein puts it:

> The process of naturalising foreign experience tends also to transform it into forms that are suitable for the national environment. The case of competition in health care – that new master idea seemingly sweeping the globe – illustrates the point well. The meaning given to this notion (inherently many-layered) has been very different in the various countries that have seemingly embraced it: if the vocabulary is international, the way in which it translated into policy remains national ... Translation often means transformation.
>
> (Klein, 1995: 98)

The next section explores this process of translation and transformation in the countries reviewed here.

Reform strategies

The case studies show that reform strategies often encompassed a wide variety of aims, relating to the equity, efficiency or effectiveness aspects of health services. Equity issues still figured prominently, particularly regarding the unequal financial burdens involved in fragmented 'risk pools' (Germany); extending population coverage of health insurance and tackling issues of adverse selection (the Netherlands, USA); tackling health inequalities in some social groups (the Maori in New Zealand). In the main however micro-efficiency concerns dominated the agenda, and in particular tackling moral hazard: the lack of incentives by consumers to restrain their demand or providers to use resources efficiently where third-party payers (whether governments, sickness funds, private insurers) pick up the final bill or most of it. As Van de

Ven *et al.* (1994) point out, conceptually third party payers carry out three main functions in health care:

- the insurance function: taking on the burden of financial risk involved in health care utilisation;
- the agency function: acting as effective agents of consumers in reducing moral hazard, being a prudent and informed buyer on their behalf, and providing information about quality of care;
- the access function: guaranteeing access to needed health services.

In most countries (the USA excepted) third-party payers have effectively carried out the first and third functions, but not the second. Improving the agency function of third-party payers has therefore been a major goal of health care reform and restructuring in many countries (although in doing so there are risks that adequate performance of the other two functions may be weakened). At the same time 'integrated' systems like Sweden and the UK wished to improve flexibility and rates of innovation in the health system or, in economists' terms, rates of dynamic efficiency.

Policy makers often had less overt agendas as well. For example, Freeman (Chapter 10) argues that the 1992 health insurance reforms in Germany represented yet another chapter in federal government's continuing 'search for control' after its failure in 1988 to reassert the capacity of 'democratic majorities to facilitate changes against the opposition of powerful organised interests' (Blüm, 1987, cited in Webber, 1991). In a very different environment, the same was true in the UK with the 1990 reforms decentralising operational control over services but continuing the long-standing Conservative policies of strengthening central controls over health authorities. GP fundholders were also 'empowered' through decentralised budgets, but their drug budgets were now effectively capped, realising a long standing Treasury ambition (Glennerster *et al.*, 1994).

'Markets', 'choice' and 'competition' are promiscuous concepts in reform documents. Similar language hides a multiplicity of meanings and intents, just as a changing discourse may symbolise changing policy directions over the reform period, with new government actors at the helm, or as different groups of stakeholders try to wrest control of the reform agenda. A good example from the UK was the renewed emphasis on health needs, public health and health 'alliances', with the publication of *Health of the Nation* in 1992 (DOH, 1992) under the influence of the Chief Medical Officer, public health physicians, some managers in the NHS Executive and the support of a more sympathetic Secretary of State. However, the softening of 'market speak' has been a more general feature in the UK, New Zealand and the Netherlands as a response to the unpopularity or unworkability of original reform concepts, and a re-emphasis on the importance of 'partnerships' and 'cooperation'.

What was the range of approaches to intervention? There are different ways to analyse such a complex range of phenomena, but in line with our primary focus – the introduction of markets and competition – it would seem useful to start with the question: were markets and competition introduced (or strengthened) in the financing of health care, the delivery of services or the way resources were allocated to providers? (See Deber and Baranek, Chapter 5, pps 81–83 for a clear explanation of this framework and the issues involved).

In terms of finance, no country substantially changed its funding systems, or introduced a private market into the financing of health care, in spite of internal debates about this in New Zealand and the UK. Countries which were already mainly funded by general taxation or social insurance remained so, while the Clinton administration proposed building on the present voluntary system of employer coverage with a compulsory mandate on all employers. At the margins there was a move towards increased user charges or co-payments particularly for drugs (UK, New Zealand, Germany, Sweden) in spite of evidence that this may be neither efficient nor equitable (Saltman and Figueras, 1996: 16–17; Carr-Hill, 1994). But in the main, financial reforms were largely directed at amalgamating separate funding streams to improve central leverage over finance, to prevent cost shifting, aid flexible deployment of services, and specify (in some cases broaden) the services that would be covered by the public system.

Instead, market incentives and competition were targeted at the service delivery system and the way resources are allocated. In 'integrated' systems (New Zealand, parts of Sweden and the UK) this required splitting purchasing and providing functions and making providers compete for the receipt of (largely public) funds through negotiated contracts. In countries where a market structure already existed it involved strengthening incentives for 'smart purchasing' (Kettl, 1993) and provider competition for contracts. The mechanisms included selective contracting with providers, performance-tied payment systems, accumulating and disseminating information on clinical effectiveness and cost effectiveness to purchasers and promoting 'managed care' arrangements (see discussion in Chapter 1, pps 6–7, also Chapter 4).

The importance of the purchasing role has been increasingly recognised, but there are big differences in who undertakes the role in line with prior historical patterns, cultural and political values (see Box 11.1).

Competition between purchasers/insurers to ensure responsiveness to users is a central feature of Enthoven's original design for 'managed competition': here the case study countries have differed in their views, with competition being extended in the Netherlands and Germany, proposed and then dropped in New Zealand. In the UK, competition between GPs for patients, both in their role as providers and (when fundholders) purchasers of secondary care, was fostered by strengthening the capitation element of their reimbursement package. The more

---

Box 11.1   Who undertakes the purchasing function?

Private corporations:	USA, Netherlands
Sickness funds:	Netherlands, Germany
Regional or local tiers of elected government:	Sweden
Primary health care districts:	Dalarna, Bohuslan counties in Sweden
Appointed regional or district public bodies:	UK, New Zealand
Private primary care physicians:	UK
Large employers:	USA

---

patients they attracted, the greater the reward. Conversely, the Clinton proposals in the USA were designed to restructure the present anarchic system of competition between insurers into a more corporatised and regulated arrangement.

The type and extent of *provider* competition seen as desirable also varied considerably, with big differences between the rhetoric of policy documents and practice. In 'integrated' systems, Saltman and von Otter (1992, 1995) have already extensively explored the differences between the main Scandinavian model of public competition between public providers which is driven by patient choice, and mixed market models of public and private providers, driven by contracts from third-party purchasers, adopted in the UK and New Zealand. Summarising the experience from different county council models within Sweden, Rehnberg (1997) concludes that direct patient choice of provider has proved to be the most powerful means of changing provider behaviour, even when this is limited to a defined range of providers with whom the purchaser has signed contracts, with real improvements in customer service (Rehnberg, 1997: 80).

In addition, the *balance* between regulation and competition varies considerably, as does the targets of regulation. On the demand side, Germany is at one extreme. While in principle introducing competition between insurers it has effectively left little room for them to compete, regulating insurance premiums, benefit packages, prices paid to providers and administrative organisations. The insurers, not surprisingly, have seriously criticised the pressures towards standardisation of their activities, and in response the Federal Minister of Health has recently proposed giving them more freedom to decide benefit packages (Schwartz and Busse, 1997: 117). The Netherlands also tried to move away from regulation to a greater reliance on competitive incentives between insurers to achieve efficiency gains, but could not overcome the technical problems of designing budgetary formulas which could maintain equity and overcome incentives to cream skimming. In the UK and New Zealand reliance on regulation increased overtime as the effects of a competitive market on the stability of providers, user access and equity became apparent.

Regulation and a range of other approaches have also been used extensively to curb pharmaceutical costs. Saltman and Figueras (1996) classify these into supply-side strategies which aim to influence physician prescribing behaviour and make them more cost conscious. These include fixed budgets, limited lists of drugs which will (or will not) be reimbursed, the use of generics rather than brand name drugs, and measures designed to improve medical practice (e.g. medical audit, clinical guidelines, budgetary incentives). Demand-side measures are aimed primarily at users and include health education programmes and cost sharing. Finally, a number of strategies are also aimed at the market as a whole, including reference pricing, controls on pharmaceutical prices and industry profits.

The health policy arena is not only shaped by the explicit decisions of ministers and governments however, but by what they choose to ignore or allowed to happen by default. The policy landscape can be decisively altered by nonintervention and lack of decision making. Private markets have been developing in this way often for major service areas for example, long-stay care services for the chronically ill and handicapped (Canada, UK), dentistry and optical treatment (UK).

Did the reformers achieve their aims?

Assessing the extent to which the reformers achieved their aims is difficult to assess. In such a complex policy sector as health care, policy goals are multiple, often ambiguous, sometimes obscure or conflicting. The aims written down in official documents may disguise less overt political or ideological agendas. Failure to achieve the former (which may in any case be rhetorical) can combine with success in achieving the latter. Reform strategies have also evolved or been reshaped over time, either from above or below, taking different directions from original intentions. The criteria of 'success' therefore changes, though this may be quietly forgotten by politicians anxious to claim credit. Some trade-offs between competing objectives are also inevitable – between equity and consumer choice, comprehensiveness and cost containment (Weale, 1988) – and evaluation of results will depend on how these trade-offs are viewed. For example, some would argue that the diversity and innovation which the reforms have promoted in Sweden, the UK and New Zealand have made services more responsive to consumers and are worth some loss of equity or higher transaction costs; others would disagree.

Nevertheless, and in spite of these caveats, it seems clear that the original *expressed* aims of reformers in New Zealand, the Netherlands, and the USA, as set out in official documentation, were not met nor implemented in the manner they were intended. This is broadly the case in the UK too, although here the evidence is more ambiguous and mixed. Germany has achieved success in controlling the pharmaceutical budget, and reforming the hospital financing system (Schwartz and Busse, 1997) and achieved reform of the insurance function to improve equity and consumer choice, but may have created new forms of perverse incentive in such a highly regulated system. Sweden has achieved real gains in efficiency, consumer choice and diversity of provision – an impressive example of the capacity of democratically controlled public services to renew themselves in innovative and efficient ways – but faces problems of longer term sustainability. Canada is still struggling to maintain a publicly funded system along prosolidarity and cost-sharing lines against intense political pressures for decentralisation by the provinces, and the pressures to allow market forces to gain a greater hold.[2]

Why did promise and performance diverge so widely? Economists might claim that politicians failed to understand how markets work and the conditions necessary for success. There are two variants of this critique. In the USA marketeers like Enthoven argue that market forces have not been given sufficient rein (Enthoven and Singer, 1994) and many American economists would agree, as witnessed by the open letter to President Clinton signed by 565 of them in 1994 criticising his proposal to have federal regulation of insurance premiums (Starobin, 1994). Other economists are far more sceptical about the benefits to be gained from introducing market incentives into health care, even with careful regulation, and argue that many of the problems highlighted by Appleby in Chapter 3, and referred to in the case studies, were predictable. Specific examples include the lack of competition for many services and the costs involved in stimulating it; information assymetries that exist between purchasers and providers in highly imperfect markets like health care, and subsequent problems of regulating opportunistic behaviour (Light, 1990; Kettl, 1993); the inability or unwillingness of individuals to act as 'informed consumers' in health care; the technical difficulties involved in appropriately risk adjusting budgets to prevent cream skimming (Newhouse, 1994; Van der Ven, 1997).

Political scientists would draw on a wider range of factors to explain why some countries were more successful than others in implementing change. A simple framework is outlined by Walt and Gilson (1994) (see Figure 11.1) which looks at the interaction between the context in which reform strategies are introduced, the process by which they are formulated, implemented and evaluated, the content of the reforms and the main actors involved.

Context includes both the macro-economic environment, discussed above, and the institutional, political and cultural environment which constrain the choices open to policy elites. It is these structural forces which, Wilsford (1994) argues, normally tie change to predetermined

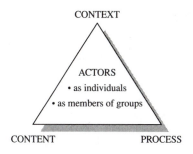

Source: Walt and Gilson, 1994

Figure 11.1 **A framework for health policy analysis**
Source: Walt and Gilson, 1994

paths and incremental policy making, but occasionally a strong conjuncture of events provides a window of opportunity to override the legacy of history and strike out on a new trajectory. For example, from an institutional perspective both the UK and New Zealand are 'strong states' (Immergut, 1992; Boase, 1994). A unicameral parliament, electoral systems which exaggerate the majority of the winning party, and a disciplined party system combine to concentrate executive power in the hands of the governing party. Structural forces are therefore less inhibiting should a radical reforming government wish to strike out on a new path, and the importance of conjunctural events is lessened although not eliminated. Hence a determined government (which had already acted to further centralise the levers of control in the health care system in the UK), could force through unpopular health reforms in spite of resistance by powerful interest groups and the opposition of the public.

By contrast the USA is a prime example of a 'weak state', in which executive power is diffused and fragmented to an extraordinary degree between federal and state governments, the two arms of Congress, the judiciary, the White House and the various executive departments, providing multiple points of access by those with interests to defend: 'American institutions are not designed to accommodate large-scale change, they are actively designed to thwart it' (Wilsford, 1994: 271). The structural hurdles faced by all presidents require an unusually strong conjuncture of events to overcome and as Mashaw and Marmor (1996) point out, these are rare and all but impossible to achieve in the case of universal health insurance. In particular the authors demonstrate the intricate interrelationships between state and federal government jurisdictions in health policy which results in the states having the political legitimacy to introduce universal health insurance but not the fiscal or legal capacity they need to do so, while federal government has the legal and fiscal muscle, but lacks the political legitimacy to carry it out.

The influence of federalism, and in particular different types of federal design, on health policy is an under-researched and fascinating area. The institutional characteristics of a federal state – which policy areas or aspects of policy (e.g. implementation) are reserved for the constituent units, how the interests of these units are represented at the national level and the extent to which fiscal equalisation is pursued – will all affect the policy dynamics and strategies of different actors and groups. Although a detailed discussion is beyond our remit, one or two examples illustrate the interaction between the two (for a fuller discussion of these points, see Pierson, 1995). As Deber and Baranek (Chapter 5) point out, Canada is an example of a federal state where specific policy areas including health care were constitutionally reserved for the provinces, and early initiatives in those spheres taken at that level. Over time this reservation of powers becomes increasingly difficult to maintain as economic interdependence and policy complexity increases (Scharpf, 1988). Central government takes action to pursue national objectives or cement national solidarity, which in Canada has been fiercely contested by the provinces. The resulting struggle over jurisdictions and political authority can rapidly turn into a full-blown constitutional confrontation (illustrated by the struggle between the province of Quebec and the federal government in Ottawa), a struggle which gets fiercer in times of economic stringency and cutbacks. The ability of the national government to iron out fiscal disparities between the provinces and use the power of the purse to enforce national standards in health care – a major component of provincial budgets – becomes less tenable when the centre is itself trying to reduce its own debts.

By contrast, in federal states where there is a *shared* jurisdiction over a particular policy domain between national government and the constituent units, policy disputes do not normally turn into full-blown constitutional crises. However, they are prone to more complex policy procedures designed to reflect the needs and interests of each tier and generally have complex decision rules to ensure these continue to be addressed in any proposals for policy reform. Shared decision making can therefore lead to 'lowest common denominator' policies which reflect the political compromises and procedural protections necessary to secure agreement. Pierson (1995) argues that this is evident in Germany, where the strong position of the Lander is assured by their control of policy implementation and their prominent role in the second chamber, the Bundesrat. The fact that the Lander regarded hospital policy as their domain, for example, was one reason why the reform of hospital financing took so long to effect. A strong conjuncture of economic and political events was necessary before central government could successfully legislate in this area in 1993 (Wilsford, 1994: 261–2).

Turning to the *processes* of reform, two points stand out from an analysis of the case studies. First, the prescriptions of economics and political science once again diverge. It is striking that the most intellectually coherent 'managed competition' reform packages in the Netherlands and New Zealand were unimplementable in practice because they ignored questions of political and administrative feasibility and acceptability. Economic rationality and political rationality diverged. Secondly, and related to this, in practice context and process are inextricably linked in a dynamic relationship. Context allowed New Zealand and the UK to take a 'big bang' approach to reform, just as it dictated a more incremental approach in the more fragmented pluralist polities of the Netherlands and Germany. In the USA Clinton's failure to take proper account of the political context was a factor in his subsequent legislative failure. The Health Security Plan was crafted with great technical virtuosity by the White House Task Force but with little sense of what would be required to get it through Congress, almost as if the President thought he was working in a parliamentary system (Ranade, 1995: 14). In Sweden a decentralised system of county council responsibility for health care allowed 'bottom up' experimentation which today provides valuable comparative data within the nation state (e.g. between county councils which implemented internal markets and those which did not, see Rehnberg, 1997).

But if context shapes process, so the process of reform can reshape context. For example, a protracted reform process (the Netherlands, USA) can lead to 'anticipated reactions' by interested parties trying to position themselves to benefit from what emerges. More subtly, as Freeman (Chapter 10, p. 189) points out, in Germany, the perpetual prospect of reform and the uncertainty that inculcates may lead health interests to restrict their profit-maximising behaviour voluntarily in fear of more restrictive legislation. The actual *failure* of legislative reform can also provoke health interests to undertake reform themselves, reshaping the context which would face policy makers in future, and probably deepening existing 'path dependencies'. The USA is a clear example of this in practice, where insurance corporations and large employers have taken on the task of cost control themselves. I will refer to the impact of this reshaping later.

The case studies also demonstrate the shifts of policy direction which have occurred during the process of implementation, and the important degree of policy learning which has taken place. In some countries this has led to a general lessening of faith in market mechanisms and a partial restoration of traditional planning and command-and-control systems. The new government in New Zealand has re-emphasised the government's role in funding *and* providing health care, and decided to remove provider competition while maintaining the purchaser–provider split. The new Labour Government elected in May 1997 in the UK has made similar noises.

The government elected in 1995 in the Netherlands has decided to remove catastrophic risks entirely from the remit of competing insurers. Services, like nursing home care and institutional care for the mentally ill and handicapped, will be planned, funded and regulated directly by central government. By contrast, the government believes that *intensifying* competitive incentives between insurers is still the best way to contain costs for noncatastrophic risks, and recent proposals will both increase the risk burdens insurers face and enforce competition through a strong procompetition policy (Van der Ven, 1997: 96).

Finally it is important to consider the scope and content of reform when looking at the failure of some reform strategies. If this is very comprehensive and wide-ranging, it risks drawing more interested parties into the frame and widens the scope for controversy and opposition (the USA, Netherlands, New Zealand). In addition the complex and esoteric nature of many of the arguments and evidence surrounding health care reform are often difficult to present simply to the public, with the risk of distortion in the media or manipulation by the lobbies. The US case provides the best example of this in practice, with millions of dollars spent on advertising and lobbying against the Clinton plan, notably and most effectively by the Health Insurance Association of America representing small and medium-sized insurers (Ranade, 1995).

Outcomes – intentional and nonintentional

Whatever the successes and failures of the reforms, they have left a legacy which reshapes the environment that policy makers face in future, both structurally and in less tangible ways, by altering attitudes, expectations and policy perceptions. This section identifies some of the major themes and similarities which emerge from the case studies.

Structural change

One theme which emerges is the considerable degree of institutional restructuring which has taken place, with complex centralising and decentralising tendencies taking place at the same time, often in the same country. On the provider side there has been considerable devolution of autonomy and a decentralisation of functions to managers in previously 'integrated' systems (Sweden, UK and New Zealand), although this has sometimes been accompanied by new forms of 'arms-length' regulation and monitoring by government bodies, as well as the incorporation of clinicians into management.

On the purchasing/insurance side, while there are instances of some decentralisation (GP purchasing in the UK, the transfer of elderly care responsibilities from the county councils to the municipalities in Sweden), consolidation and 'regionalisation' would better describe the general picture, with functions devolved down from the national level and up from the local. This has normally been done to create larger and more powerful purchasing bodies capable of exerting greater leverage on providers, better risk management and service restructuring. In some cases these changes in roles and authority have been accompanied by constant debate and tension about the appropriate role of central government. Examples include:

- mergers between country councils in Sweden;
- mergers between health authorities in the UK (which are likely to continue under the Labour Government);
- consolidation of sickness funds and private insurers in Germany and the Netherlands;
- the establishment of regional health authorities in New Zealand;
- the creation of regional (though still small) administrative bodies in Canada, although the tensions between provincial and federal government are another aspect of this phenomenon.

An associated phenomenon is the growing corporatisation and consolidation of health care institutions generally, either through horizontal mergers (sickness funds, private insurers, provider chains) or through vertical integration between insurers and providers. This is most marked in the USA where the prospects of health care reform based on managed competition and managed care has led to the growth of giant corporate chains (Salmon, 1995). One result of this is a change in the importance of investor-owned for-profit institutions at the expense of not-for-profits, but even when not-for-profits survive they are forced to behave increasingly like their for-profit competitors (Salmon, 1995: 17).

Nevertheless, ownership status *does* influence behaviour. Schlesinger and Smithey (1994: 70) argue that for-profit provider institutions are more likely to select patients on the basis of ability to pay, to locate in areas of higher incomes, to avoid offering services used most by the poor, and to screen patients for insurance status. Even though the policy environment is different, there are lessons here for countries where facilities are still mainly publicly owned or who rely extensively on the not-for-profit sector. Some influential voices in the UK, for example, have argued that fears about the eventual privatisation of NHS trusts are misplaced. The real issues are how the insurance/purchasing function should be discharged, and the maintenance of government funding and universal access: 'It is this, far more than the privatisation or not of trust hospitals, that affects whether patients will still have access to appropriate and necessary services' (Ham, 1994: 10). However, this view may at best be a half truth, overestimating the regulatory abilities of governments, and underestimating the costs and the power of commercial incentives and practices to dissolve, like acid, the cultural values of public service and social solidarity.

Trust managers have already proved to be sharp entrepreneurs, increasing their share of private operations from 11 to 15 per cent between 1988 and 1995. This is expected to rise to 20 per cent as more private pay beds are opened (Whitehouse, 1997). NHS trusts also operate private beds more efficiently with occupancy rates averaging 70 per cent compared to 40 per cent in the independent sector, and subsequent lower costs passed onto the consumer (Whitehouse, 1997). If trusts are privatised, the temptations to concentrate even more on fee-paying patients at the expense of meagrely reimbursed public patients must surely increase.

Changes in the pattern and location of services

Service delivery systems are being reconfigured to take account of technological developments in medicine and informatics, which allow more services to be delivered out of hospitals in primary health centres and clinics and in the patient's home. Progress is often dependent on removing budgetary and organisational barriers which prevent the flexible use of monies and staff between primary, secondary and community services, and there are many examples in the case studies of the ways in which these are being tackled. The growing importance of primary health care as the major focus for the health system, which may be reversing two hundred years of history in which hospitals have dominated the scene, is another noteworthy trend. This is turn has implications for the role, location and functions of the hospital sector, but as the UK has discovered, closing or 'rationalising' hospital services is politically very difficult to achieve, whether undertaken by traditional top-down planning mechanisms, or in response to competitive pressures.

Changes in the balance of health care interests

This unprecedented degree of structural change has created new groups of stakeholders with interests to defend, or restructured the power and influence of existing groups. In very broad terms and at the risk of oversimplification, the power of medical interests has declined in relation to that of managers (and health economists!) as doctors are subject to growing pressures to make their practice more transparent and accountable, through the use of explicit contracting mechanisms, managed care and the growth of clinical guidelines, and so on. The extent to which these impinge on the status and autonomy of doctors differs considerably in different countries (in the USA McKinlay and Stoeckle, 1994, have argued that it is 'proletarianising' the profession, see also Salmon, 1994; North, 1995) but the trend is unmistakeable. Meanwhile, attempts to 'empower' users through the reforms, whether through expanding choice or enhancing voice have had mixed results (see below).

Effects on users

The introduction of market principles into the provision of publicly provided health systems has been accompanied by a change of language.

'Patients' have been turned into 'consumers' and encouraged to expect more choice and improved quality of service. In general these expectations have been, at best, partially met in the UK and New Zealand. Only Sweden appears to have achieved considerable success in improving choice of provider (with users having the formal right to choose a provider anywhere in the country), and reducing waiting times (with a maximum waiting time guarantee of three months, among other quality improvements).

In the 'public contract' systems of the Netherlands and Germany and in the USA and Canada, consumer choice was always a strong value, but here as in New Zealand and the UK the case studies provide examples of growing restrictions on choice and coverage for users from the spread of managed care developments and more explicit rationing procedures. (In the USA 75 per cent of working Americans are now covered by Health Maintenance Organisations or other forms of managed care, Bransten, 1997). Ironically, the Clinton proposals would have guaranteed consumers a choice of at least three health plans, but as large employers and insurers take on the job of cost containment themselves after the failure of the legislators, choice and competition are being squeezed out of the market. As Woolhandler and Himmelstein (1994) point out, as the USA 'gallops towards oligopoly', the only choice consumers will have is to go to Giant HMO 'A' or Giant HMO 'B'.

The case studies also showed that support for publicly funded systems had held up well but is clearly under strain and conditional on performance. In that respect the translation of 'patients' into more demanding 'consumers' may have fuelled the very cost pressures governments are anxious to contain. Saltman (Chapter 9) argues the imperative of seeking supplementary forms of community-based finance which do not imperil equity and solidarity, and points out that current attempts to devise more explicit rationing procedures for public systems, notably in Sweden, the Netherlands, and New Zealand, whatever principles they are based on, would inevitably mean reductions in service for poorer people from which richer groups could buy themselves out.

The changing role of the state

The role of the state in publicly funded systems has changed but not declined. In formerly integrated systems 'government by contract' in complex quasi-market relationships has been added to (rather than replaced) direct hierarchical forms of control. In practice government agencies have less experience in managing these relationships and still lack sophisticated theories about what incentives work in gaining the compliance of providers. In addition, for government to act as a 'smart buyer' in such a highly imperfect market as health care requires substantial prior investment in its capacity to specify the services it needs and monitor the quality of the contractor's performance, investment which is often neglected. It must then suffer the consequences of ineffective and inefficient purchasing (Kettl, 1993).

It is also far more difficult to steer these complex networks of public, quasi-public and private organisations in the same direction, leading to a loss of strategic control. This is a particular problem in the UK, where the fragmentation of the 'local state' has been carried furthest. Under the impetus of 'new public management' doctrines and the ideological crusades of Mrs Thatcher, the traditional local power centre – elected local government – has lost influence and functions to nonelected single purpose agencies and commercial interests (Cochrane 1993). Today this seems a perverse step to take when it is increasingly acknowledged that complex social problems (like the poor health status of socially deprived groups, for instance) require a coordinated multi-agency attack under strong local leadership, and the broad public health strategies promoted by the World Health Organisation's Health for All 2000 find increasing intellectual acceptance throughout Europe. Paradoxically, in countries like the Netherlands and Germany, where a pluralistic 'public contract' system already existed, the state is trying to gain more effective control through stronger central regulation, more powerful purchasing authorities, and so on.

Conclusions and lessons

Comparative analysis reveals a substantial degree of convergence between states in the perceived problems and burdens facing health care systems, and in the language used to express them, but policies are formulated and implemented in divergent national contexts. The case studies reveal a wide range of constraints (including ideological beliefs) which:

• limit the policy options considered and the agenda of reform, and – just as significantly – what is not on the agenda and remains as rhetoric;
• affect the scope of the reforms, and whether radical or incremental change is pursued;
• shape the compromises made in the course of implementation.

It is also clear that though the language of reform is the same, similar words have multiple meanings. Underlying concepts can differ profoundly and one important task of comparative analysis is to illuminate these differences and prevent too superficial generalisations being made. Nevertheless, with nearly a decade of international experience to draw upon, there are increasing attempts to generalise from the experience of introducing market incentives in health care (see, for instance, Saltman and Figueras, 1996; Ham, 1997; OECD, 1994b) and draw lessons on what has worked and what hasn't. Maybe some of the most important lessons concern the process of lesson drawing itself. It is obvious now that managed competition was seized on as a quick fix to solve diverse problems of health systems in the importing countries, with remarkably little evidence as to its feasibility in its country of origin or transferability to very different institutional and cultural contexts. Now, as faith in competition as a panacea recedes, other panaceas are being seized on just as uncritically. 'Evidence-based medicine', managed care and the shift from hospitals to primary care settings have a role to play in containing costs and improving the effectiveness and accessibility of services, but they are far from being panaceas or quick fixes, can generate unanticipated problems and – like managed competition itself – can be implemented in many ways, with different benefits and costs (for a fuller discussion see Maynard, 1995).

If policy makers are to improve their capacity to draw lessons from international experience they must be able to distinguish the circumstances in which a particular policy innovation succeeded or failed and therefore whether there is any point in trying to transplant it into foreign soil (Klein, 1995). This requires strengthening the capacity for critical analysis and the testing of alternatives. Klein argues that 'cross-national learning is rather like a multi-ring circus with different actors performing in each of them' (1995: 7). Politicians and civil servants, managers and doctors, political scientists and economists, all have different languages, perspectives and timeframes, ask different questions and seek different answers. It is only through this clash of perspectives and confrontation of ideas that real learning can take place. At the same time governments need individuals who can act as 'policy translators' to demystify disciplinary jargon and communicate their insights to practical politicians and managers.

The deliberate introduction of dissenting views into policy circles, through for example think-tanks or policy units attached to the core executive, helps to attack tendencies to 'group think' among government elites, and exposes ideas to stronger critical testing. Devil's advocates are necessary even if they are uncomfortable to have around. In this respect it is encouraging to see some of the imaginative appointments of outsiders in the new Labour Government in the UK and plans to reinstate something like the Central Policy Review Staff, a think-tank within government, with an independent brief to 'think the unthinkable' on long-term strategic issues, introduced by Edward Heath in 1970 and abolished by Mrs Thatcher 10 years later.

To argue that greater rationality in the policy process is possible (and desirable) is not to argue 'the end of ideology'. Clearly governments work within different value frameworks to attain their strategic objectives, but should at least make these explicit to provide clear benchmarks against which policy alternatives can be tested, and the results can be evaluated. One of the chief criticisms made of the UK and New Zealand experiments with markets in health care was the failure to articulate strategic goals (or the lurch from one to another), and the way in which competition was treated as an end in itself rather than the means by which other goals could be achieved.

At a systems level, the policy lesson which bears repeating over and over again is that financing health care mainly through private insurance is neither equitable nor efficient, and the USA is clear witness to this. Insurance overheads and a competitive market has made the US system the most costly in the world, yet it still fails to cover the health care needs of millions of its citizens. Even Enthoven (1990) agreed that the only lesson the USA has for Europe in this respect is what to avoid (for a particularly pungent analysis see also Evans, 1997). Yet we are more sceptical than other recent commentators that this lesson has been well learnt (see, for instance, Ham, 1997). The fiscal and economic pressures which triggered health care reform in the first place have not disappeared, and private markets are developing by attrition and default as much as conscious design.

Whether the market will go on rising in health care, or whether it is yesterday's story, is still an open question, dependent on how health care fits into the political economy and political and social culture of each country. The reasons lie in the twin face of health care: as a core function of the welfare state and an industry of massive proportions. The power and size of the 'medical-industrial' complex in the USA for example is now as great as that ascribed to the 'military-industrial complex' in the 1960s (Salmon, 1995). The reshaping of the health care state is inextricably caught up in the wider welfare and industrial restructuring precipitated by the emerging dynamics of global capitalism and the struggles for national competitiveness. The balance between market forces and welfare values in health care will depend on how these struggles are resolved.

Notes

1   Salter (1995) estimates that even in the UK with the most substantial degree of government involvement, 52 per cent of NHS expenditure is spent in the 'private' sector, if this is defined as goods or services privately owned or private produced (GPs, pharmaceuticals, general dental and opthalmic services, supplies and equipment, etc.).

2   Ironically, given the former status of Canada as a role model for many in the 'single-payer' reform camp in the USA (see for instance Himmelstein and Woolhandler, 1992) Deber and Baranek (Chapter 5) note how politicians in some Canadian provinces have become late enthusiasts for markets! Perhaps they have most to learn from the failure of other countries' market experiments.

References

Boase, J.P. (1994) 'Institutions, institutionalized networks and policy choices: Health policy in the US and Canada', *Governance*, **9**(3): 287–310.

Bransten, L. (1997) 'The Americas: US health care costs', *Financial Times*, 25 March, p. 8.

Campbell, C. (1995) 'Does reinvention need reinvention? Lessons from truncated managerialism in Britain', *Governance*, **8**(4): 479–504.

Carr-Hill, R. (1994) 'Efficiency and equity implications of the health care reforms', *Social Science and Medicine*, **39**(9): 1189–1201.

Cochrane, A. (1993) *Whatever Happened to Local Government?*, Buckingham: Open University Press.

Department of Health (1992) *The Health of the Nation*, Cm 1986, London: HMSO.

Enthoven, A. C. (1990) 'What can Europeans learn from Americans? In *Health Systems in Transition: The Search for Efficiency*, OECD Social Policy Studies, No. 7, Paris: OECD.

Enthoven, A. C. and Singer, S. (1994) 'A single payer system in Jackson Hole clothing', *Health Affairs*, **1**: 81–95.

Evans. R.G. (1997) 'Health care reform: Who's selling the market and why?', *Journal of Public Health Medicine*, **19**(1): 45–9.

Fukuyama, F. (1992) *The End of History and the Last Man*, London: Hamish Hamilton.

Glennerster, H., Matsaganis, M. and Owens, P. (1994) *Implementing GP Fundholding: Wild care or Winning Hand?*, Buckingham: Open University Press.

Ham, C. (1994) 'Private versus public is not the issue: Hospital ownership is a diversion', *The Independent*, 24th August, 10.

Ham, C. (1997) *Health Care Reform*, Buckingham: Open University Press.

Himmelstein, D. and Woolhandler, S. (1992) *The National Health Program Chartbook*, Cambridge, Massachusett: Harvard Medical School.

Immergut, E. (1992) *Health Politics: Interests and Institutions in Western Europe*, New York: Cambridge University Press.

Kettl, D. F. (1993) *Sharing Power: Public Governance and Private Markets*, Washington D.C.: The Brookings Institute.

Klein, R. (1995) *Learning from Others: Shall the Last be the First?* Four Country Conference on health care reforms and health care policies in the United States, Canada, Germany and the Netherlands Rotterdam February.

Light, D. (1990) 'Learning from their mistakes', *Health Service Journal*, **99**(1548): 1–2.

Marmor, T. R. and Maynard, A. (1994) *Cross-national Transfer of Health Policy Ideas: The Case of 'Managed Competition'*, International Political Studies Association Conference, Berlin August 1994.

Marmor, T. R. and Plowden, W. (1991) 'Rhetoric and reality in the intellectual jet stream: The export to Britain from America of questionable ideas', *Journal of Health Politics, Policy and Law*, **16**(4): 807–12.

Mashaw, J.L. and Marmor, T. R. (1996) *'Can the American state guarantee access to health care?'*, in P. Day, D. M. Fox and E. Scrivens (eds) *State, Politics and Health: Essays for Rudolph Klein*, Oxford: Blackwell.

Maynard, A. (1995) *Don't Confuse Me with the Facts, Stupid!*, in Four Country Conference on Health Care Reforms and Health Care Policies in the U.S. Canada, Germany and the Netherlands, Amsterdam, February.

McKinlay, J. B. and Stoeckle, J. D. (1990) 'Corporatization and the social transformation of doctoring', in J. W. Salmon (ed.) *The Corporate Transformation of Health Care, Part 1: Issues and Directions*, Amityville, NY:
Baywood.

Newhouse, J. (1994) 'Patients at risk: Health reform and risk adjustment',
Health Affairs, **11**, Spring, 132–46.

North, N. (1995) 'Alford revisited: The professional monopolisers, corporate rationalisers, community and markets', *Policy and Politics*, **23**(1): 115–25.

OECD (1988) *Ageing Populations: The Social Policy Choices*, Paris: OECD.

OECD (1987) *Financing and Delivering Health Care*, Paris: OECD.

OECD (1992) *The Reform of Health Care: A Comparative Analysis of Seven
OECD Countries*, Paris: OECD.

OECD (1994a) *New Orientations for Social Policy*, Social Policy Studies 12,
Paris: OECD.

OECD (1994b) *The Reform of Health Care Systems: A Review of Seventeen
OECD Countries* OECD: Paris.

Pierson, P. (1995) 'Fragmented welfare states: Federal institutions and the development of social policy', *Governance*, **8**(4): 449–78.

Ranade, W. (1995) 'US health care reform: The strategy that failed', *Public
Money and Management*, Summer: 10–16.

Rehnberg, C. (1997) 'Sweden', in C. Ham (ed.) *Health Care Reform*, Buckingham: Open University Press.

Ridley, F. J. (1996) 'The new public management in Europe: Comparative perspectives', *Public Policy and Administration*, **11**(1): 16–29.

Saks, M. (1991) 'The alternatives to medicine', in J. Gabe, D. Kelleher and G.
Williams (eds) *Challenging Medicine*, London: Routledge.

Salmon, W.(ed.) (1994) *The Corporate Transformation of Health Care, Part
11: Perspectives and Implications*, New York: Baywood.

Salmon, W. (1995) 'A perspective on the corporate transformation of health
care', *International Journal Of Health Services*,**25**(1): 11–42.

Salter, B. (1995) 'The private sector and the NHS: Redefining the welfare state'
Policy and Politics, **23**(1): 17–30.

Saltman, R. and Figueras, J. (1996) *European Health Care Reforms: Analysis of
Current Strategies*, Copenhagen: WHO Regional Office for Europe.

Saltman, R. B. and von Otter, C. (1992) *Planned Markets and Public Competition*, Buckingham: Open University Press.

Saltman, R. B. and von Otter, C. (1995) *Implementing Planned Markets in
Health Care*, Buckingham: Open University Press.

Scharpf, F. W. (1988) 'The joint decision trap: Lessons from German federalism and European integration', *Public Administration*, **66** :239–78.

Schlesinger, M. and Smithey, R. W. (1994) 'Nonprofit organization and health
care', in T. R. Marmer (ed.) *Understanding Health Care Reform*, Newhaven,
Connecticut: Yale University Press.

Schwartz, F. W. and Busse, R. (1997) 'Germany', in C. Ham (ed) *Health Care
Reform*, Buckingham: Open University Press.

Starobin, P. (1994) 'Flunking economics?' *National Journal*, 3 December, 581–6.

Taylor-Gooby, P. (1996) 'Paying for welfare: the view from Europe', *The Political Quarterly*, 67: 116–26.

Taylor-Gooby, P. (1997) 'European welfare futures: The views of key influen-
tials in six European countries on likely developments in social policy', *Social Policy and Adminstration*, **31**: 1–19.

Van der Ven, W. (1997) 'The Netherlands' in C. Ham (ed) *Health Care Reform*, Buckingham: Open University Press.

Van de Ven, W. Schut, F.T. and Rutten F. F. (1994) 'Forming and re-forming the market for third-party puchasing of health care', *Social Science and Medicine*, **39**(10): 1405–12.

Walt, G and Gilson, L. (1994) 'Reforming the health sector in developing countries: the central role of policy analysis', *Health Policy and Planning*, **9**: 353–70.

Weale, A. (ed) (1988) *Cost and Choice in Health Care*, London: King's Fund.

Webber, D. (1991) 'Health policy and the Christian–Liberal coalition in West Germany: The conflicts over the health insurance reform 1987–8', in C. Altenstetter and S. Haywood (eds) *Comparative Health Policy and the New Right*, London: Macmillan.

Whitehouse, E. (1997) 'Pay beds pose a problem for the big three insurers', *Financial Times*, 23 May, Special Supplement, p.2.

Wilsford, D. (1994) 'Path dependency, or why history makes it difficult but not impossible to reform health care systems in a big way', *Journal of Public Policy*, **14**(3): 251–83.

Woolhandler, S. and Himmelstein, D. U (1994) 'Galloping towards oligopoly: Giant HMO 'A' or Giant HMO 'B'', *The Nation*, 19th September, 285–8.

INDEX